"Suzanne Friedman's teaching style and her books reveal a generous and firm willingness to make her enthusiasm for qigong accessible to others."

—Dr. Antoine Delaly, acupuncturist, medical hypnotist, and qigong practitioner in Lausanne, Switzerland

"Friedman's in-depth studies and prolonged practice of Taoist meditation has enabled her to understand aspects of qigong practice that are not usually uncovered by Western academics and practitioners. Given such a perspective, her book is the first of its kind—lucid, original, and practical."

—Grandmaster B.F. YeYoung, Taoist Inner Alchemist and former University Professor of Chinese Philosophy and Arts in China

"Lao Zi, ancestor of Taoism, once said 'the only reason that we suffer hurt is that we have bodies; if we had no bodies, how could we suffer?' How to achieve 'no body'? Begin with the qi practice now! This book will show you how."

—Dr. Xu Hongtao, doctor in the qigong department at Xiyuan Hospital in Beijing, China

"The techniques in this book could change your life for the better. Get going and you'll see for yourself."

—Joseph M. Helms, MD, president of Helms Medical Institute

"Finally, a book that demystifies qigong and makes it accessible to a large audience. If you have ever had second thoughts about trying qigong, this book will point you in the right direction. I have waited a long time for a book like this to give to my students and patients."

—Fia Hobbs, MMQ, LMT, BodyCareConsultants in Stockholm, Sweden

"Suzanne Friedman's book is a unique and important work that will enable readers to harness qigong to significantly improve their health. Clearly and beautifully written by one of the most respected authorities on the subject, *Heal Yourself with Qigong* unlocks the many secrets of this powerful healing system from the East."

—Dermot O'Connor, author of *The Healing Code*

Heal Yourself with Qigong

Gentle Practices to Increase Energy, Restore Health, and Relax the Mind

SUZANNE B. FRIEDMAN, L.AC., DMQ (CHINA)

NEW HARBINGER PUBLICATIONS, INC.

Distributed in Canada by Raincoast Books

Copyright © 2009 by Suzanne B. Friedman
New Harbinger Publications, Inc.
5674 Shattuck Avenue
Oakland, CA 94609
www.newharbinger.com

Cover design by Amy Shoup; Text design by Amy Shoup and Michele Waters-Kermes;
Acquired by Jess O'Brien; Edited by Kayla Sussell

Printed in the United States of America

Library of Congress Cataloging-in-Publication Data

Friedman, Suzanne B.
 Heal yourself with qigong : gentle practices to increase energy, restore health, and relax the mind / Suzanne B. Friedman.
    p. cm.
 Includes bibliographical references.
 ISBN-13: 978-1-57224-583-9 (pbk. : alk. paper)
 ISBN-10: 1-57224-583-2 (pbk. : alk. paper)
 1. Qi gong. I. Title.
 RA781.8.F7488 2009
 613.7'148--dc22

                              2008052238

FSC
Mixed Sources
Product group from well-managed
forests and other controlled sources

Cert no. SW-COC-002283
www.fsc.org
© 1996 Forest Stewardship Council

11   10   09

10   9   8   7   6   5   4   3   2   1

First printing

For Becca,
la princesa

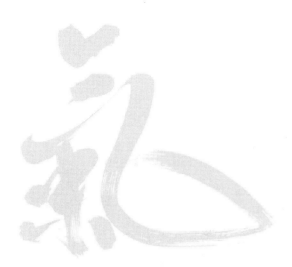

CONTENTS

CHAPTER 5
Restoring Physical Vitality

CHAPTER 7
Calming Your Spirit

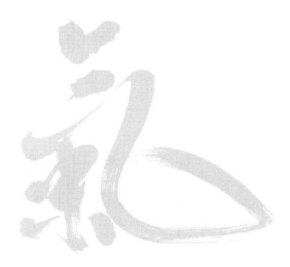

FOREWORD

I trained in acupuncture in France in the mid-1970s. Each morning before seeing patients my teacher and I spent an hour going through a sequence of tai chi chuan postures. I had spent a year learning the sequence in Berkeley, where Master Lee taught only one small move per lesson, per payment. He claimed to be a "master of a rare northern style" of tai chi, and was the spearhead of a wave of tai chi "masters" immigrating to California and the United States.

We felt well stretched and virtuous as we approached the day's patients. I tried to sustain this rhythm when I started my own practice, but within a few years I reluctantly admitted that I had never tapped into the rush of vitality, tranquility, or spiritual connection that I had been promised. Indeed I was well stretched, but bored, and the virtuous feeling no longer justified the time it took to do the sequence. So I abandoned tai chi for exercise that I felt was better suited to my age: jogging, swimming, biking, and I have continued with the latter two—increasingly intermittently—through my middle age.

As the wave of tai chi masters transformed into a tsunami of qigong masters, I tried again. Qi is, after all, the stuff we push and pull around the body with our acupuncture needle patterns. Same experience: a transient feeling of virtue, some new stretches for an older and less flexible body, but still requiring too much time for its promised and largely unrealized benefits.

Then I met Dr. Suzanne Friedman, a *true* master of medical qigong, who understands the daily challenges of striving to keep a balance among body, psyche, and spirit while living in the real world. Her approach to qigong is refreshingly straightforward, honest, and generous. She embodies the same attitude I found so appealing in my teachers in France: an enthusiasm for every student to understand and learn what she has to teach, a clarity and openness in offering the information, and an encouragement for students to personalize and integrate the techniques according to their individual interests and needs.

That's what *Heal Yourself with Qigong* is about: making qigong work in your life, for you, and making it available as well to those you influence, in a style remarkably easy to assimilate and put into practice. And it's not boring.

Dr. Friedman starts with an overview of the history and theoretical foundation of qigong, nicely sprinkled with encouraging scientific references. She then moves quickly into the fundamental tenets of practice, very directly and in easy-to-understand language. She next provides general techniques for cultivating physical well-being, and then offers techniques appropriate for specific medical problems. In the final chapters she addresses emotional balance and spiritual integration. It's a tour from theory to practice, from body to emotions to spirit, that reveals details not available elsewhere, at least not without years of apprenticeship.

The integrative programs that Suzanne and I have developed for physician graduates of my acupuncture courses have been remarkably successful. Her medical qigong exercises facilitate a rapid and comfortable assimilation of the advanced acupuncture approaches I enjoy teaching. Qigong gives the theoretical material an experiential foundation, which locks the information more securely into the students' psyches. Feedback from our students is enthusiastic, for both personal and professional applications.

Suzanne Friedman teaches what she practices: showing practitioners and patients how to heal themselves with qigong. She takes seriously the Daoist tradition of empowering patients to stay well by taking attentive care of all aspects of their being. Her book opens doors that have been kept closed by teachers who pass on their learning to only a few students at a time. This book not only demystifies qigong, it makes it into a lively and appealing daily habit well worth acquiring.

I have wondered briefly how my life might have been different had Dr. Friedman been around thirty years ago to transform my disillusionment with tai chi chuan. Only briefly, because there's still plenty for me to learn and gain as I genuinely feel and move qi. The living sensation transcends simply feeling virtuous. It's feeling vital, balanced, whole. Thank you, Suzanne Friedman, for making *Heal Yourself with Qigong* available to all of us.

—Joseph M. Helms, M.D.
President, Helms Medical Institute
Founding President, American Academy of Medical Acupuncture
Author, *Acupuncture Energetics*, and *Getting to Know You*
August 2008, Berkeley

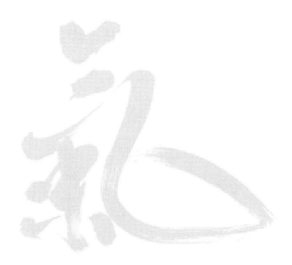

ACKNOWLEDGMENTS

To begin at the beginning, I was blessed to be born into a wonderful family. Thank you to my folks for their unwavering support, and to my sister Jolie for being exactly who she is.

I am eternally grateful to my qigong teacher, Grandmaster YeYoung, for taking me under his wing and, perhaps most importantly, for walking the walk.

Special thanks go to my Breath of the Dao clinic patients and my students at the Acupuncture and Integrative Medicine College (AIMC) in Berkeley, who are my most valued teachers on a daily basis. The lessons of my past teachers, Dr. Jerry Alan Johnson, Shifu Alex Feng, Dr. Xu Hongtao, Dr. Robert Johns, Pamela Olton, and Brian LaForgia, continue to inspire me and inform my every decision in the clinic.

I must acknowledge the top-notch staff at New Harbinger, who made this project such a pleasure. Thanks to Jess O'Brien for finding me and for sharing my passion, to Jess Beebe for her improvements, and to Kayla Sussell for her sharp eye.

Everyone who knows me knows that I could not have done this, and everything else I do, without Becca.

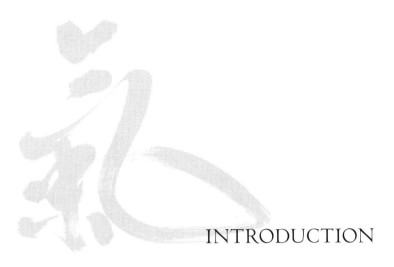

INTRODUCTION

THE POWER OF
ANCIENT TECHNIQUES IN
A MODERN WORLD

How are your energy levels? Do you have enough energy to sail through all of your daily responsibilities? Or do you crash at a certain time of day? If you do crash, do you get a second wind? These questions are a part of every routine Chinese medical examination. I have been asking these questions in my clinic every day for years now, and the answers might not surprise you. But what might surprise you is the direct correlation between the answers and the person's overall mental and physical health.

How much energy you have determines so much on a day-to-day basis; in fact, your energy levels practically shape your life. They are a direct reflection of your vitality as well as an indication of how well or poorly you are aging. In terms of chronological time, we are all growing older at the same pace, but how quickly our bodies or minds break down from the wear and tear of aging is an entirely separate issue.

The therapeutic energy exercises in this book have been practiced in one form or another for hundreds, if not thousands, of years. What is unique about this book's presentation of qigong (pronounced "chee gong") is that it is designed for busy, tired, working people who have little time to spend on themselves. In short, people who are looking for and can use a little more balance in their lives. For that reason, I've included only those exercises that produce powerful and almost immediate results.

Some of these exercises come from hospitals that practice Chinese medicine; others are those that I've either taught or prescribed to my patients. They are all time-tested potent techniques, which either calm the mind and body or boost energy, both of which have the effect of slowing down the aging process. It can take as little as five minutes of practice to feel the benefits of these qigong exercises. You do not have to memorize difficult, lengthy exercise regimens. Nor do you have to buy new clothes or fancy equipment. If you have just five minutes, you can pick and choose any one exercise and do it at any time, depending on what your health goal is.

When I say that qigong can transform your life, I speak from experience. My own transformation story began back when I was a litigation attorney who didn't believe in the power of anything as subtle as qigong or visualization techniques. Actually, in the interest of full disclosure, I must admit that I was initially introduced to qigong in 1989, when I was living in Japan.

While living in Japan, I tried my hand at meditation and found that I was a lousy meditator. I couldn't sit still comfortably for more than ten minutes, and I couldn't stop my mind from racing from one thought to the next. The more I tried to quiet my mind, the more unruly it seemed to become. Nonetheless, I knew intuitively that I needed something to balance out my type A lifestyle.

One day I came across a flyer in English for a weekend workshop in something called "Taoist yoga." I was intrigued and figured that I couldn't be any worse at whatever Taoist yoga was than I was at meditation. I went to the workshop, and the entire morning was spent practicing ridiculously easy qigong exercises. (It turns out that qigong used to be called Taoist yoga back in the 1970s and '80s). I couldn't understand how these exercises could possibly benefit me when I wasn't even breaking a sweat. Moreover, the visualizations seemed too corny and too New Age for me to take seriously. I didn't stay for the afternoon session, nor did I return the following day. Instead, I wrote it off as a complete waste of time and money, and laughed about the experience with my friends.

The following year I entered law school as planned, and I started my own law firm almost exactly one year after I graduated. When I was an attorney, I prided myself on my ability to multitask; for example, it was not unusual for me to prepare for a court case while eating lunch and simultaneously talking on the phone with a client or opposing counsel. I specialized in writing appeal briefs (written arguments) for my clients as well as for other lawyers in California and Texas.

I regularly overextended myself by taking on more cases than I could handle, and to meet deadlines I routinely sacrificed quality for speed. This was accepted by other lawyers, because they conducted their own practices in the same manner. It was part of the profession's "culture" to accept as many cases as came in through the door, as each case meant more money. By all measures, I was a success. I had a thriving law practice and I won a number of appeals cases, the decisions for which were published in the law books and became case law.

Along with my success came chronic insomnia, anxiety, digestion issues, sugar crashes that affected my moods, and an irregular heartbeat when I was particularly stressed. Routinely, I would get to my office by 6:30 A.M. to prepare for 8:30 A.M. hearings. I ate breakfast (always a sugary scone or muffin and a double cappuccino) in my car on the way to the office. Lunchtime was never spent just eating lunch; instead I would concurrently write motions or briefs, or I would work on a case or two as I quickly scarfed down my food. I clearly remember always rushing from one place to the next, or from one task to the next. Each day was a nonstop whirlwind of activity.

When I got home after work, I crashed hard. Back then I wasn't a napper, and I rarely got a second wind. I went to bed exhausted but was frequently unable to sleep. If I did fall asleep, I would wake around 3:00 A.M. full of anxiety about the briefs I had to write or the hearings I had to attend the next day. Anxiety became my default mental state. This went on for years, and I can honestly say that I saw nothing wrong with how my life was going; I merely accepted the consequences of what I thought was necessary to succeed in my chosen field.

A few years later, I went on a family vacation to the Canyon Ranch Spa in the Berkshire Mountains of Massachusetts. On a whim, I chose to get an acupuncture treatment instead of the usual massage. I told the acupuncturist that my legs and back were sore from the hiking, running, kayaking, and racquetball I had squeezed into the day before. (Back then I thought that if you worked hard, you should also play hard.) I was worried because the following day would be the second day after heavy exercising, which is usually when I feel most sore. To my surprise, I woke up the next day feeling oddly refreshed and entirely without muscle soreness. I was blown away by the power of one twenty-five-minute treatment.

When I got back to San Francisco, I bought a couple of books on Chinese medicine. Then I bought a few more. The more I read, the more I wanted to learn. Chinese medicine presents a medical model based on wellness; one in which doctors are paid to keep their patients healthy, instead of getting paid only when their patients become ill. I was particularly intrigued with its focus on balancing body and mind, and the belief that the body and the mind cannot be seen as separate entities.

I knew that my own daily mental stress was negatively affecting my physical body, but I had no clue that I could harness my mind to positively affect my body. In truth, I didn't believe it was possible for the mind to affect the body back then, but I was completely intrigued by the idea, and so I kept reading book after book on Chinese medicine. At some point during that time I had a sudden realization: It was like a lightbulb going off over my head, just like in a cartoon. I suddenly knew what I was supposed to do with the rest of my life. Within six months of my acupuncture treatment at the spa, I enrolled in pre-med classes, and then I entered a four-year program at the American College of Traditional Chinese Medicine in San Francisco.

While in Chinese medicine school, I still ran my law office. I would often put on a suit in the morning, go to court, change clothes, and then go to class (or the reverse). Ironically, my life became even more hectic while I was trying to learn balance. I met my acupuncture mentor right after I began school, and he reintroduced me to qigong and encouraged me to practice it. Memories of Taoist yoga in Japan came flooding back to me, but I trusted this man, and I began practicing the qigong exercises he taught me.

Even though I was working full-time and going to school full-time, I found I had plenty of energy. I learned that ancient Chinese medicine doctors considered self-healing to be the highest form of medicine, and that they showed their patients qigong exercises so that those patients could take an active role in their own healing and wellness. I was already experiencing the energy-boosting benefits of qigong practice, and I found that I was able to focus my mind more clearly on whatever I was doing. I also realized that I could learn how to share qigong with my future patients. So while still enrolled in Chinese medicine school, I enrolled in a separate medical qigong therapy master's degree program, and I followed that with a doctorate in medical qigong therapy after completing my clinical hours at the Xiyuan Hospital in Beijing, China.

I treated patients and taught qigong exercise classes while at the Xiyuan Hospital. I saw how doctors from all of the different wings sent their patients to the qigong classes, regardless of their illnesses or injuries. Patients routinely told me that after all else had failed, it was their daily hour of qigong that helped them feel better or even healed them from whatever their ailment happened to be.

That was many years ago, and since then I've taught thousands of people how to perform and practice qigong exercises. I have personally witnessed students and patients heal from physical and psychoemotional illnesses using qigong as one of their main healing tools. I've had many people come up to me to tell me about healing "miracles" they have experienced due to their qigong practice. Today, I no longer underestimate visualization techniques and gentle exercises that don't make you feel as though you had just finished running a marathon.

The Daoist theories that underlie Chinese medicine teach that the simplest things can also be the most profound, and that less is more. It can take years to break unhealthy patterns and to shake the belief that change is impossible. The beauty of the qigong approach is that you simply start from where you are. Tiny steps can still take you where you want to go; you just need to dedicate some of your time to yourself, which is a form of self-respect and love. Let's face it: when you have more energy and your moods are well-balanced, you are also more pleasant to be around.

Happily, the anxiety, insomnia, and other problems that I dealt with when I was an attorney are long gone. I have learned how to balance work and rest, and I regularly practice the "KISS principle," which means "keep it simple, stupid." Now when I eat, I just eat. If I am tired midday, I take a twenty- to thirty-minute nap and I wake up refreshed. It took a while for my chronic anxiety to abate, but it did; and I sped up the process with qigong visualizations that balance my emotions. I still begin each day at my clinic with at least thirty minutes of qigong, which ensures that I will be focused and have the energy I need to be the best doctor I can be.

I have come to understand that some of the deepest and most effective healing is not found at a doctor's office or a hospital, but rather from inside ourselves. Our bodies are designed for self-healing, and we are capable of both boosting and blocking that ability. It takes literally only minutes a day to calm the mind and restore and revitalize our energy, and this book will show you how to do that. These exercises continue to work wonderfully for me, and I know they will work for you.

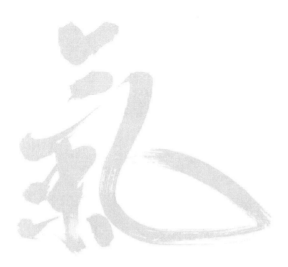

CHAPTER 1

QIGONG DEMYSTIFIED

Although qigong is a common form of exercise in China, it is just starting to take off here in the United States. These days you can find more and more people practicing qigong and tai chi in public parks all around the country. When I first started practicing, there were only a handful of qigong videos available on the market, and let's just say that the quality of those videos left something to be desired. Now, you can easily find hundreds of good quality videos, DVDs, and even qigong classes with a simple Web search. (See my website at www.medicinalqigong.org.) What was once a secretive practice passed down by masters is now available to everyone, and today we can all benefit from qigong's increasing popularity.

Once you have started a regular qigong practice, you will begin to feel the health benefits of the exercises, but it is also good to know the theory behind what you are doing.

Accordingly, in this chapter I've tried to answer some of the most common questions people have about qigong. Knowledge is power, and the more you know about qigong, the more powerful your practice will be.

WHAT IS QIGONG?

Qi (pronounced "chee") is the life-force energy of the body, which is responsible for our vitality. *Gong* means skill or work. Qigong is therefore the practice of accumulating and cultivating vital life-force energy in the body. (Note that qigong is sometimes written as "chi kung.")

Qigong is composed of three essential aspects: (I) physical exercises, (2) meditation and visualization, both of which are considered the practitioner's "mental intention," and (3) breathing exercises. Qigong was developed into a systematic healing art to preserve health and vitality during the Era of the Warring States in China (from sometime in the fifth century BCE to the unification of China in 221 BCE). Excavations done in 1973 discovered a qigong exercise chart from 168 BCE, which shows forty-four movements, or exercises, along with commentaries on their therapeutic benefits (Peng 1990). Doctors from that time, who were then shamans, practiced and taught qigong to their patients. Today, Chinese medicine doctors continue to work in that lineage's disciplines. Because qigong has been practiced for centuries, the exercises that work have remained; those that did not work were not passed on. Thus we are lucky to have more than two thousand years of qigong "clinical trials"!

Qigong, the focus of this book, is a main branch in traditional Chinese medicine. There are three different schools of qigong: martial, medical, and spiritual. *Medical qigong* is the cultivation of energy specifically to preserve and restore health. It consists of techniques that relax and integrate the mind and body and strengthen the body's tissues and organ functions. It is a self-healing therapy that gives the person practicing qigong a greater degree of control over the aging process. Qigong practice has been linked to improved circulation, reduced stress, lowered blood pressure, reduced chronic pain, and improved immune function (Sancier 1996b).

Qigong exercises involve a combination of proper posture, proper breathing, and guided intention. *Proper posture* allows the body's energy to flow more freely through the body. *Proper breathing* calms the nervous system while providing the body's cells with more oxygen to use as fuel. *Guided intention* involves focusing the mind on a specific goal, such as calming anxiety or increasing energy flow to the organs of the digestive system for improved digestion.

HOW WIDELY USED IS QIGONG?

For thousands of years, millions of people in China have benefited from qigong practices and have used it to heal disease and maintain health. In fact, Chinese doctors can specialize in medical qigong as their main area of expertise for healing patients in hospitals and clinics. Here in the United States, tai chi, a martial arts branch of qigong, has been steadily growing in popularity.

Chinese medicine schools in the United States now require their students to learn qigong exercises, and currently these practicing and future acupuncturists are spreading the word. In addition, studies that demonstrate the power of a regular qigong practice are attracting the attention of the mainstream medical community (Curiati 2005). As a result, more and more people are discovering the healing and rejuvenating benefits of qigong, which unlike tai chi is specifically geared toward self-healing. Today, qigong is becoming one of the fastest growing exercise systems in our country, as evidenced by the hundreds of qigong videos currently available to the public.

WHAT ARE THE BENEFITS OF QIGONG?

The effects of qigong practice include prevention and healing of disease, relief from stress, improved physical strength, improved mental focus, improved sexual function, and spiritual enrichment. One of its main benefits is its ability to slow down the aging process.

One review of various clinical studies concluded that qigong has positive effects on the following markers: hypertension (blood pressure); mortality and stroke; levels of superoxide dismutase (SOD) called "the anti-aging enzyme" because it scavenges free radicals that cause cellular damage; sex hormone levels; cardiovascular function; cancer; and senility (Sancier 1996a).

ARE THERE SCIENTIFIC STUDIES ON QIGONG?

Yes, there are many scientific studies on qigong. In addition to the scientific findings referenced above, researchers have demonstrated that the practice of qigong has positive effects on blood viscosity, bone density, endocrine gland function, asthma, immune function, serum lipid levels (cholesterol), sexual function, the incidence of strokes (it reduces the risk), as well as a host of other benefits (Sancier and Holman 2004).

Qigong exercises have been prescribed with great success in Chinese hospitals, and numerous clinical trials have demonstrated the healing effects of long- and short-term qigong practice. There are at least two studies that demonstrate qigong reduces chronic pain and enhances mood states in elderly patients (Myeong et al. 2001; Tsang et. al. 2003).

Although I don't conduct scientific studies, I've personally seen significant physical and emotional benefits in patients ranging from twenty to eighty years old. It is not unusual for patients to report their surprise about how much better they feel within a week or two of practicing qigong. In fact, after almost every qigong seminar I teach, I receive numerous e-mails from participants either telling me how much better they feel or that they showed an exercise to someone else who now feels better as a result of practicing that exercise.

SHOULD YOU TALK WITH YOUR DOCTOR ABOUT BEGINNING QIGONG PRACTICE?

All doctors know that moderate exercise such as qigong has a beneficial effect on the heart, blood circulation, and joints. They are now becoming more aware of the beneficial effects of deep breathing and meditation on the nervous system, mood, cognitive function, and memory. Nevertheless, if you have a specific ailment that limits your range of motion or strength, or any chronic illness or health issue, you should always check with your doctor before beginning any new exercise regimen.

I routinely encourage my patients to check in with their doctors to chart the effects of their qigong practice on such markers as cholesterol, weight, blood sugar (fasting glucose), blood pressure, and mood.

HOW LONG SHOULD YOU EXPECT TO PRACTICE QIGONG BEFORE YOU SEE RESULTS?

Practicing just five to ten minutes a day will have immediately measurable effects on your body and mind. The increase in qi (energy) flow improves blood circulation, lubricates the joints, relaxes the nervous system, and dispels stress from the muscles and the mind.

The longer you practice consistently, the deeper the effects. Similarly, the beneficial, anti-aging effects of qigong increase and accumulate as the years pass. Ideally, you will develop a *daily* qigong practice, as a few minutes a day is far more beneficial than thirty minutes done every three or four days.

As I said in the introduction, originally, I did not believe that anything as subtle as visualization or slow-moving exercises could have any effect whatsoever on my health or mental state. Nonetheless, I began a regular qigong practice that continues to this day. It did not take very long for me to notice that my emotional state and physical stamina had started to improve. I began with ten minutes a day, every day. It took me a while to build up to my current practice, which is thirty to forty-five minutes each morning. The beauty of qigong is that after you practice regularly for some time, you will want to practice even more.

IS QIGONG A RELIGIOUS PRACTICE?

Qigong is not affiliated with any religious beliefs or systems, nor does it conflict with any religious beliefs or systems whatsoever.

Chinese medicine holds that each person has or is comprised of "three treasures." These are the mind, body, and spirit. Some qigong exercises, meditations, and visualizations involve connecting with your spirit, or true self, to help accelerate the healing process. Others involve the cultivation of a sense of inner peace and a deeper connection with your spiritual self. Qigong practice can be molded to incorporate a particular spiritual or religious belief, but only if that is what you desire.

The last chapter of this book is entitled "Calming Your Spirit." Perhaps it will be helpful if I describe here what I mean by "spirit." When I talk about the spirit, I am referring to your higher self, and to the person within you that you aspire to become. These exercises and meditations focus on relaxing your body and mind so that you can experience and harness a feeling of calm and tranquility that will, over time, carry over into the rest of your day.

CAN YOU PRACTICE QIGONG WHILE ENGAGING IN OTHER FORMS OF EXERCISE?

Absolutely. Qigong practice does not interfere with other forms of exercise, such as working out at the gym, jogging, or doing yoga, Pilates, or any other form of movement. In fact, I have taught qigong to numerous athletes and martial artists as a way to enhance their athletic performance, endurance, and strength. Most of these athletes report better focus and greater stamina as a result of practicing qigong before a competition.

I encourage people who work out hard to balance their strenuous physical activity with qigong. Qigong will help the body and mind to relax and recover, and it helps keep the joints lubricated, which prevents or lessens chronic pain. Moreover, we all need some aerobic (heart pumping) exercise; walking briskly for just twenty to thirty minutes a day counts. Walking gets you out in nature, and it has been shown to alleviate depression.

It is said that moving the body helps move the mind out of the feeling of "being stuck," and I have seen people's depression lift without medication when they combine good walks with a regular qigong practice.

IS IT POSSIBLE TO DO TOO MUCH QIGONG?

Every now and then someone will ask me, "How much qigong practice is too much?" This is typical of our culture, where we feel that if a little is good, more must be better. This can be true with qigong, but only to a degree. There is no need to practice for hours a day, and when people report doing so, I often find that is because they are using their practice as an avoidance technique or an escape.

The purpose of qigong is to help you to engage more fully and healthfully in life. If you do too much of anything, you cannot find balance. Practicing up to an hour a day is more than sufficient. You can do two twenty-minute sessions, or one longer session, per day. I recommend that you start with only five to ten minutes a day because it is easier to set aside such a small chunk of time every day, no matter how busy your lifestyle or daily schedule.

The advantage of starting slowly is that as you begin to feel the effects, your desire to practice increases naturally. When that happens, there is no need to force yourself to practice and, in fact, forcing yourself to practice rarely leads to an organic, long-term practice. Take an honest look at your schedule and plan accordingly. It is best to set yourself up for success, rather than setting goals that will be hard to achieve. Sometimes more is just more; it is not better.

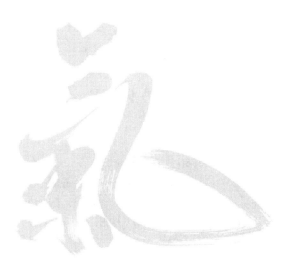

CHAPTER 2

GETTING STARTED:

THE SIMPLE BASICS

There are a few simple guidelines when starting a qigong practice. Luckily, they are easy and intuitive. Adding something new to your daily routine can be difficult, but if you plan it well and then follow through with your plan, you will reap the physical and emotional benefits of your qigong practice in no time at all. However, as with any exercise routine or martial art, there are ways to practice that will keep you safe while helping to accelerate improvements in your skill level and stamina.

START WHERE YOU ARE: SET YOURSELF UP FOR SUCCESS

The most common recipe for failure is to set a goal that is beyond your reach. If you have a partner and a child or children—and you work full-time—that leaves room for little else, not to mention time for yourself. First, take a realistic look at your daily routines; don't aim for thirty minutes a day if you don't have that kind of time. Start where you are by doing what you can; no more—but no less.

It's important to keep in mind that the practice of qigong will give you more energy and help you balance your emotions, and can help with any physical aches and pains you might have. You will find that when you feel better and have more energy, you will be a more pleasant person to be around, and this can improve the quality of all of your relationships. These few minutes devoted to your qigong practice, away from your responsibilities, will have far-reaching effects on your daily life, and the people in your life will appreciate the changes they see.

When to Practice

In the beginning, even though it may be hard to find the time to practice, as previously stated, it is better to practice for a few minutes a day, five to seven days a week, than for thirty minutes a day but only twice a week. Be kind to yourself when you start, and be sure to set yourself up for success. Pick a specific time to practice each day and set aside that time slot exclusively for your qigong practice. If you wait for an opening to appear in your daily routine, it may never happen. You must be willing to take a proactive approach. Think about how you brush your teeth every day. Because you have been doing it for so long, brushing your teeth has become an effortless habit. The same thing will happen with practicing qigong—if you choose a consistent time slot in which to practice.

You can find exercises that work well for you at night, just before you go to bed, or those that work well for you in the morning, just before you go to work. Or you could take ten minutes out of your lunch break. Perhaps you have some time after dinner every evening? There may even be a lull at work each day when you can take five to ten minutes to try some of these exercises.

The bottom line is that daily practice is more important than where or when you practice.

When Not to Practice

There are times when you should not practice qigong. For example, it is not a good idea to practice when you are emotionally distraught, as it is difficult to focus your mind and relax when you are agitated or upset. If you are exhausted or have a cold, I recommend that you take a nap rather than practice. Do not push yourself to do more than your body will allow. More is not always better, so start slowly and build from there. Furthermore, you should never practice when under the influence of alcohol or drugs.

Although five to ten minutes may not seem like a lot of time, it will likely lead to longer practice sessions once you begin to feel the difference from doing the qigong exercises and meditations regularly. I like to think of the time I practice qigong as a special sacred time distinct from the rest of my day. It is the time when I get to focus on nothing but my own mental, physical, and spiritual well-being. I pay no attention to anything that might have happened before I begin, and I don't think about what I have to do when I'm finished. Instead, I turn my attention to the immediate moment, where all that is required of me is calmness, being relaxed, and mental focus.

Turning your attention to the present moment encourages you to become more grounded and focused, and these characteristics will spill over into other aspects of your life. You'll find that you are able to concentrate better, think more clearly, and have more control over your emotions after you have practiced qigong for some time. (The length of time needed to experience these benefits varies.)

Right now would be a good time to take a realistic look at your schedule to figure out when you will be able to incorporate your qigong practice into your daily routine.

Where to Practice

You can practice the exercises you'll find in this book anywhere. Many or most of them can be practiced at your desk, in a chair, and even lying down. This makes it even easier to put this book to good use anytime you have a few minutes to devote to yourself.

Ideally, you will find one or two places that will become your dedicated healing space. You may have a quiet and well-lit room in your home. Or you can devote a corner in your bedroom just to your practice. You might hang calming pictures, create an altar with personal objects that have meaning for you, play soothing music, or burn incense to make the room your special practice space. It is also important to let your family or roommates know that you are not to be disturbed during your qigong time.

If it is easier to practice at work, then use a particular time of day to create the feeling of a healing space by not answering the phone, closing the door, or even just closing your eyes. You can play a particular piece of music on your computer, MP3 player, or stereo that you listen to each time you do your qigong, so that over time whenever you hear that piece, it will put you in a calm, relaxed mood. If your office has carpeting, perhaps you can take off your shoes. That will help to put you in the zone so that you can really focus on your qigong exercises instead of on your work tasks during the time you set aside to practice.

I practice when I arrive at my clinic every morning, exactly one hour before my first patient is scheduled. I used to play a particular CD every time, but now I prefer to practice in silence. I take off my shoes, watch, and eyeglasses, and I go to the same spot every time. The phone is turned off so it can't interrupt me. When I'm finished, I put on my watch and glasses, turn the phone on, and make myself a cup of tea minutes before my first patient arrives. This ritual has completely eliminated my old habit of rushing around in the morning and feeling stressed about what lies ahead that day. Instead, I feel energized and centered and ready to be present for my patients and whatever else the day may bring.

Think of where you would like to start your qigong practice. What can you do to that area to make it special? What do you need to do to create a space and a time that will make it both easy and inviting to cultivate your own well-being every day?

What to Wear

Unlike yoga, qigong does not require that you wear special clothing when you practice. That being said, your clothing should not be so tight that you cannot move freely. However, there are some exercises and meditations in this book that require minimal or no movement, and for them it doesn't matter what you wear, since they are based more on intention than posture.

If you choose to practice the exercises standing up, you should wear flat shoes that provide good support. Sneakers, flat dress shoes, and bare feet (weather and location permitting) are all fine. *Warning:* Don't buy those cute black tai chi shoes that you see in videos! They give no support and can even lead to foot pain and bone spurs.

Keep in mind that any loose-fitting comfortable clothing is the best qigong "uniform," be it dress or casual clothing, or even pajamas.

Practicing Alone vs. Practicing with Others

As with dieting and other forms of exercise, having a partner helps you stick to the regimen you create for yourself. Many of my students and patients have told me that when they have someone else with whom to practice, they practice more consistently. This may not be practical if you have a very busy schedule, but it is something you may want to consider.

Furthermore, it is a widely held belief that the more people practice together, the more each person feels the qi during the practice. When a group of people are moving their bodies in the same way and focusing their minds on the same task, it creates a qi field that invigorates and energizes each individual's practice. Anyone who has practiced qigong in a group will report this, even beginners.

Having said that, what is most important is that you practice consistently, and if you can't find consistent partners, it is better to practice alone.

CHAPTER 3

ESSENTIAL PRACTICE COMPONENTS: POSTURE, BREATH, AND INTENTION

Posture, breath, and intention are the three essential components of qigong practice. They are the elements that differentiate qigong practice from mere exercise or calisthenics. Every qigong exercise has its own proper posture, breathing technique, and mental focus. When you follow them correctly, you will be able to feel the benefits of that exercise more quickly. Note that I believe this chapter is the most important one in this book, because without proper posture, breath, and intention, you are not practicing qigong!

PROPER POSTURE

Correct physical posture and weight distribution prevent tension and injury, and allow energy to flow freely throughout your whole body. If you stand or sit in an uncomfortable position, it is difficult to focus your mind on the exercise or meditation. Chinese medicine views pain as the result of a blockage of qi (energy) and blood flow, and proper posture ensures that the exercises are comfortable and your practice remains pain free.

Correct posture regulates the heart and calms the mind by enhancing qi and blood circulation. This makes it easier to lead the flow of qi downward to reduce stress. Stress, anger, and anxiety have an upward-moving energetic quality, which often leads to head-aches, neck and shoulder tension, and even jaw clenching. Qigong helps send energy down from the head toward the feet, resulting in a more relaxed body and calmer mind.

There is a relaxation sequence that occurs when practicing qigong. First, your muscles relax, followed by the tendons and ligaments relaxing, then the nerves, and finally the bones. You can think of your physical body as a vessel into which energy can be added and then circulated.

Qigong practice positions your body in a way that maximizes the flow of energy to smooth out any blockages that have been causing pain or discomfort, while strengthening the body itself. If you should experience pain during any of the exercises, lessen your movements; for example, don't turn or bend too deeply. Or you can change your positioning to avoid pain. If there is pain, there is *no* gain; so stop just before the point of feeling any pain with any exercise that may be challenging for you.

When practicing qigong, you may begin to feel the enhanced qi flow through various areas of your body. Many people experience bodily sensations such as heat, tingling, vibration, or a sense of fullness. When qi flows through your nerves, you may experience an energetic current or electric-like surge through your body or arms or legs.

There are descriptions of the proper ways to stand or sit during your qigong practice below. When you follow the instructions for the basic standing posture, which is called *wuji* posture, you will notice your muscles, knees, and back becoming stronger. If you are unable to stand for too long, you can practice most of the exercises and meditations from a seated position. The masters say that standing builds qi quicker, but as I noted earlier, it is best to start where you are.

Wuji Posture: How to Stand

The following is a beginner's list for proper standing posture, which is called *wuji* posture. *Wuji* posture is the foundation for all *dynamic* (moving) and *quiescent* (static) standing exercises. This posture maximizes relaxation and the flow of qi.

1. ## Stand with Your Feet Flat

    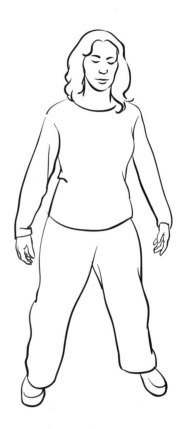

    "Stand with your feet flat" means that you should distribute your weight evenly through your feet, rather than have it unevenly distributed on your heels, toes, or the sides of your feet. Your legs are separated as wide as your shoulders' distance apart and your toes should point forward.

    Your toes should softly grasp the ground to keep your body firmly rooted yet relaxed. Rigid or tense feet disrupt the flow of qi from the earth into the body.

    While training, your feet may vibrate or feel hot. This is a normal reaction to correct postural training and is beneficial because it can help dissolve any calcium deposits accumulated in the bottoms of your feet—the soles and heels.

2. ## Bend Your Knees

    Your knees should be slightly bent and facing the same direction as your feet. Never bend your knees past your toes. Try to align the knees directly over your feet, if possible and comfortable. Many people develop knee problems from various forms of exercise because they bend their knees too far forward or allow their knees to twist. Relaxing the knee joints increases the qi and blood flow through the legs.

3. Relax Your Lower Back

Relax your buttocks, back, waist, and hips. Try to reduce the curve in your lower back by tucking your *coccyx* (tailbone) down. Keep your upper body straight. Your buttocks should be gently tucked in to help strengthen your spine. You may also imagine a heavy weight hanging from your coccyx. As the weight pulls down, tilt your *sacrum* (the last bone at the bottom of the spine, which directly connects to the pelvis).

4. Tighten Your Anal Sphincter

Gently tightening the anal sphincter seals the gathered qi in the body. Although the anal sphincter is held closed, it is important that the perineum and buttocks remain relaxed. Initially, you may find it difficult to use abdominal breathing while keeping your anus tightened. Be assured that it will rapidly become an unconscious reflex after some practice.

5. Relax Your Chest and Arms

Your shoulders should be gently pulled back and then down, without puffing out your chest. When you breathe, your chest should stay relaxed with minimal movement. When your chest and back are without tension, your heart and lungs are able to function more efficiently, and circulation of both qi and blood is improved.

Your elbows are slightly bent and held at the sides of your body with your palms facing the outsides of your thighs. Move your arms slightly away from your body so that your elbows are very slightly bowed out.

6. Suspend Your Head and Tuck In Your Chin

Visualize your body as if it were suspended by a string connected to the crown or top of your head. This will elongate your spine and slightly tuck your chin in. Slightly tucking your chin in and stacking your vertebrae on top of one another facilitates qi and blood flow through your spine and brain. Feel your spine elongate with each breath. Check each part of your body to ensure that all your muscles are relaxed.

7. Close Your Eyes for Inner Vision

It is easier to feel or guide inner qi circulation with your eyes closed. Your eyes remain closed during meditations and visualizations.

However, when practicing dynamic (movement) exercises, your eyes stay slightly open with a soft focus. Keeping your eyes open will keep your body balanced.

8. Touch Your Tongue to the Upper Palate in Your Mouth

When your tongue touches the upper palate behind your teeth, it connects two major *meridians* (acupuncture channels) like a circuit and enhances qi circulation in the front and back of your body. Your lips are gently closed and your teeth are gently touching. This seals in the qi and prevents it from leaking, as does tightening the anal sphincter.

Seated Posture

You can practice many of the exercises and meditations from a seated position. If you are sitting in a chair, sit toward the front edge of the chair with both of your feet firmly planted on the ground. Your legs are slightly separated, and your palms rest on your thighs. Try to minimize the curve in your back by tucking your buttocks under and sitting upright, as though your head is suspended by a string. Tuck in your chin slightly to lengthen the back of your neck.

You can sit on a cushion placed on the floor as well, if that is more comfortable for you. Try to sit so that your buttocks are slightly higher than your knees. This will form a triangle between your knees and your lower abdomen, which establishes a firmer connection to the energy field of the earth.

PROPER BREATHING

Because relaxed breathing directly calms the nervous system, qigong masters have always placed a great deal of importance on the breath. In fact, breathing is your one direct link to your nervous system. It is the means by which you can control the fight-or-flight response of your sympathetic nervous system and activate your parasympathetic nervous system to respond with what has been called both the "feed-and-breed response" and the "rest-and-digest response."

When you are in a stressful state, your breathing becomes rapid and shallow and your heartbeat accelerates. Quick, shallow breathing makes it harder for your lungs to do their job, which is to supply your body with oxygen and remove waste and toxins from your bloodstream. In addition, when you focus your mind too intensely on a particular task (as is normal at work), your muscles begin to contract and become tense, and your breathing is limited. Also, a sedentary deskbound job can lead to frequent slouching, which also limits the lungs' ability to expand fully.

Deep inhalation increases the flow of lymph fluid from other parts of the body into the thoracic duct of the lymphatic system, and *exhalation* creates a suction effect that enhances the veins' ability to empty the duct; therefore, proper breathing helps keep the body's extracellular fluids clean and circulating properly. This, in turn, helps prevent disease within the lymph and organ systems. Deep breathing also lowers blood pressure, massages the abdominal organs, and stimulates *peristalsis* (the movement of food through the digestive tract).

Qigong breathing, also called diaphragmatic or abdominal breathing, has an immediate calming effect on the nervous system. By slowing down your breath, you slow down your mind and relax your muscles, and stress and tension melt away. It is the easiest, cheapest, most portable stress-relieving tool available to us.

Qigong breathing will also recharge your body's energy levels. Deep abdominal breaths saturate your blood with extra oxygen, which is one of the quickest and most effective ways to cleanse your bloodstream and deliver energizing oxygen throughout your body. Oxygen is the most vital component in the production of *adenosine triphosphate* (ATP), the compound that transports chemical energy within cells. (Biologists call ATP "the energy currency of life.") Thus, the more oxygen you breathe in, the more energy your body can produce for healthy daily living.

Most people push out their chest when they inhale and collapse the chest when they exhale. Their abdomen barely moves. I call this the "stress breath." Qigong breathing draws in air using your diaphragm—not your chest cavity. Instead of filling your chest, you push out your abdomen on the inhale to draw more breath into your lungs, as I will soon describe. As a result, your lungs fill more efficiently, supplying the cells of your body with more oxygen and with the production of more energy. At the same time, qigong breathing produces a calming effect on your mind and body.

You can practice qigong breathing anytime, anywhere. You can do it while commuting to work, waiting in line, or watching television, and when you simply need to recharge your body and mind. This is the type of breathing that you should do with every exercise and meditation in this book.

Qigong Breathing: Step-by-Step

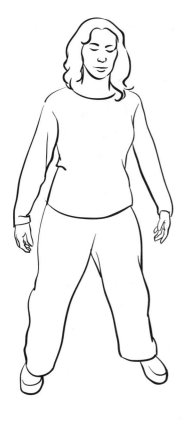

1. Stand in *wuji* posture or sit comfortably on a chair or cushion. Breathe only through your nose and keep your mouth closed.

2. When you inhale, push your belly out to pull breath into the bottom of your lungs. The key here is to be sure that your chest barely moves: All of the movement should come from your abdomen. Fill your lungs from the bottom to the top while pushing out your belly.

3. When you exhale, pull your belly in to help expel the air and waste products from your lungs. Again, your chest should barely move.

4. Breathe slowly and smoothly. Relax your entire body.

5. If you are doing qigong breathing alone (as opposed to breathing with an exercise or meditation from this book), add the visualization of inhaling vitality and energy into your body, and exhaling tension and stress from every muscle and cell. With every in-breath, visualize your body being filled with vitality and energy. With every out-breath, visualize every muscle and every cell of your body relaxing and releasing tension.

If you have trouble with qigong breathing at first, you can practice by lying on your back and placing a heavy book on your belly. When you inhale, stick your belly out and push the book up. When you exhale, pull your belly back in and the book back down. *Optional:* Keep one or both hands on your chest to see if you can help reduce its movement.

PROPER INTENTION

Proper intention means the active use of imagination, visualization, and affirmation during a meditation or exercise. All three affect and alter the creative subconscious mind, which in turn reprograms the body. Intent leads the mind (thought), and the mind leads the qi (energy). We use imagination and visualization to help focus the mind to guide the flow of qi through intended pathways, and to enhance the benefits of a qigong exercise or meditation.

The Chinese say, "When you root the mind, the spirit becomes open to ten thousand voices." Here, the "mind" means your analytical rational mind. By giving your mind a visualization task, you relax your body and become able to feel more from the exercises. You also enhance your ability to tap into your spirit, or your true self (the ten thousand voices). Concentration and thought are both catalysts for chemical reactions in the body. Concentration causes energy to congeal and solidify. Focused intention and visualization calm the emotions and reduce the perception of discomfort in the body. This means that we can use our minds to slow and deepen our breathing, which will then calm our emotions and relieve stress, tension, and anxiety.

Using intention to guide energy is not just wishful thinking. Research has confirmed that focusing the mind on positive images affects a wide variety of physiological functions, including heart rate, blood pressure, respiratory patterns, oxygen consumption, brain wave rhythms, gastrointestinal function, hormone and neurotransmitter levels in the blood, and the immune system. In fact, guided imagery, intention, and visualization therapy are used in hospitals and clinics worldwide to treat conditions from headaches, nervous stomachs, and anxiety to cancer (Rossman 2000).

The exercises that follow include visualizations that enhance the benefits of the exercise while tasking the mind to stay present and involved in the process. When I first began practicing qigong, I often ignored the visualization instructions because I didn't think they were important, or because I couldn't keep my mind focused for more than a few minutes at a time. Since then, I have come to believe that the visualizations are the most important aspect of qigong practice. They help to cultivate a sense of mindfulness and of being in the present moment. This leads to greater control over your emotions and a deeper sense of inner calm. I cannot overemphasize the value of relaxed but focused mind concentration during qigong.

At first, it may be difficult to keep your mind focused while you practice qigong. But I am happy to report that this skill is easily developed through consistent practice. Like everything else in life, the more time you dedicate to cultivating an ability, the faster you acquire that ability.

Whatever you decide to do, and whenever you decide to begin, be gentle and patient with yourself. Keep tabs on your physical, mental, and emotional states over time; and check in with yourself regularly. You will notice a very subtle but undeniable shift taking place at the deepest levels of your being as qigong becomes easier and easier. Now let's get started!

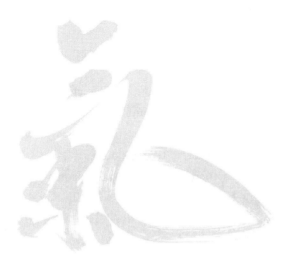

CHAPTER 4

INSTANT ENERGY

BOOSTERS

This chapter contains exercises that specifically work to boost energy levels, mental focus, and physical well-being. They are designed to get the qi and blood moving to revitalize your body for a quick energetic pick-me-up. These exercises are the perfect substitute for that midafternoon cup of coffee, can of soda pop, or sugary snack.

There can be many reasons for your energy levels not being as high as you would like. You may simply be tired from a chronic lack of adequate sleep. Or your body may be tired because it doesn't get the fuel it needs from the food you choose to eat. Chinese medicine calls this state a *qi deficiency*, meaning that your energy levels are depleted.

On the other hand, you may be tired due to daily stress and tension, chronic emotional upset, or physical pain. All of these conditions block the flow of qi; Chinese medicine calls this state a *qi stagnation*. In these instances, your energy is not low, it is just blocked, and moving the qi you already have can help boost your energy levels tremendously.

The exercises in this chapter have been shown to help regardless of the reason your energy levels are low. The key is to remember to practice them when you need an energy boost, which, ironically, is usually the time you feel as though you don't have enough energy to practice. I encourage you to get into the habit of practicing any of these exercises just before you start to feel too tapped out to practice. They will help you get going in the morning, and prevent late afternoon crashes. Pick and choose a few that immediately appeal to you. Trust your intuition, as your body has its own innate intelligence. Over time you will find yourself drawn to certain exercises over others. Go for it!

1. Cleanse the Qi: To Calm Your Mind and Get Your Energy Moving

Cleanse the Qi is an ancient qigong exercise currently used in modern Chinese hospitals to lower blood pressure and reduce stress and tension. As stated earlier, stress and anxiety have an upward-moving energetic quality, something like a feeling of "butterflies" that begins in the stomach and works its way up to the heart and mind. This exercise will get your energy flowing, ground and root your emotions, and send your stress and tension down into the ground. *Caution:* Because of its downward-moving nature, this exercise is contraindicated for pregnant women.

It is called Cleanse the Qi because you will gather the calm energy around you, wash it through your entire body, and then send it down and out through your feet, taking your stress and tension with it. I like to begin and end my qigong practice with this exercise. I use it to help ground my thoughts and to stop me from thinking about what I was doing before I began my qigong routine. It helps to move me into the present moment and signals the beginning of that special time of each day dedicated to my own healing and well-being.

Cleanse the Qi looks like a very simple exercise, but it may be challenging to incorporate abdominal breathing with your movements. Many of my students find it helpful to start by practicing deep breathing while standing in wuji posture without moving. Once you are comfortable breathing properly while standing, add the arm movements of this exercise into your routine.

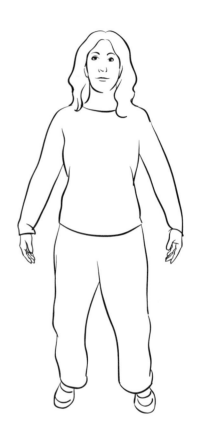

1. Begin *wuji* posture by standing with your feet apart just about the width of your shoulders. Keep your knees slightly bent and your toes facing forward. Tuck your tailbone under to minimize the curve in your lower back. Tuck your chin in slightly and line up your head over your torso by standing straight. Relax your eyes with a soft gaze. Allow your hands to hang naturally by your sides, with the palms facing the outsides of your thighs.

2. Once you are standing comfortably, begin qigong breathing. Push out your abdomen on your inhale and pull it back in on the exhale. Take a few deep, slow breaths to ready yourself.

3. On an inhale, raise your arms out to your sides with your palms facing the earth until your arms are at your shoulders' height. Visualize gathering the energy around you as if you were gathering a bright white light.

4. While still inhaling, turn your palms up to face the sky and continue to raise your arms over your head. Continue to visualize gathering the energy around you like a bright white light.

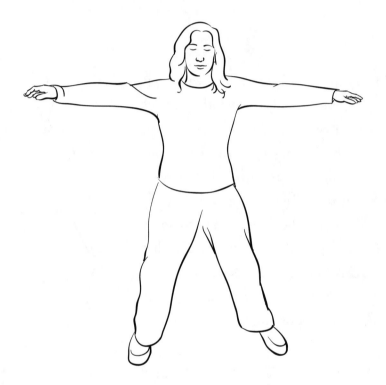

5. Exhale slowly once your arms are almost straight up with the palms facing each other, and then slowly bring your hands down the front of your body, with your palms facing the earth and your fingertips pointing toward each other. Visualize the bright, white light energy flowing through your entire body, cleansing all stress and tension as you send the energy back down, deep into the earth.

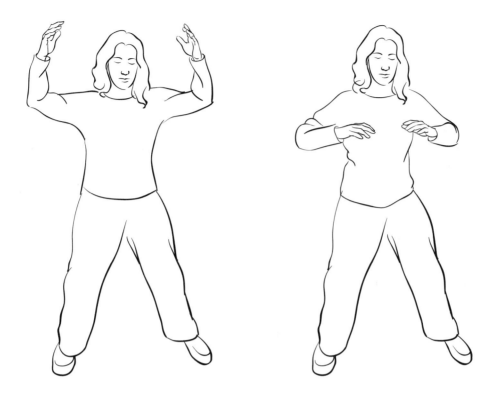

6. Repeat by inhaling and bringing your arms out to your sides and over your head. Then exhale as you bring your arms down the front of your body with your palms facing the earth.

Begin with two minutes and work up to five minutes twice a day.

Cleanse the Qi is one slow fluid movement that follows the breath. There is no stopping during or between repetitions. The combination of breath, movement, and visualization is what makes this a potent qigong exercise, so it is essential that you use the visualization of gathering energy and sending it down through your body as you practice. The more slowly you can practice Cleanse the Qi, the more soothing it is.

2. Stretch and Support the Sky: To Energize Your Whole Body and Relax Muscle Tension

Stretch and Support the Sky is the perfect quick pick-me-up. It gets your blood flowing while stretching your muscles and meridians. (The *meridians* are the acupuncture "highways," or channels, that conduct energy to and from different areas of your body.) This is also the exercise of choice if you sit in front of a computer all day and suffer from neck, shoulder, or wrist tension. Stretching your arms upward gives your lungs more room to take in a bigger breath, which means more oxygen is provided as fuel for your body's cells.

1. Stand in *wuji* posture. (You can also do this while sitting, but your lower body will miss the stretch it receives when you stand.)

2. Place the backs of your hands on top of your head with your palms facing the sky and the fingertips of both hands pointing toward each other.

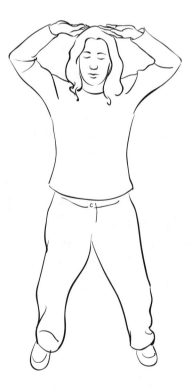

3. Inhale into your belly, and then exhale and stretch your arms directly up above your head. At the same time that you begin to raise your arms, rise up on the balls of your feet to stretch your legs. Keep your palms parallel with the ceiling as you stretch upward until your elbows and knees are no longer bending.

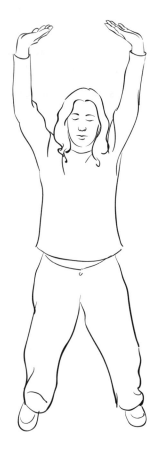

4. Exhale, and lower your arms and hands back to the starting position while coming back down to flat feet.

5. Inhale, and raise your arms directly overhead while rising up on the balls of your feet. Stretch and elongate your entire body. Keep your head facing forward.

6. Exhale, lower your arms, and come back down onto your feet.

7. Repeat at least 9 times if you can, fewer if you can't.

You may find that your shoulders are too tight to raise your palms directly up over your head. Don't push to make this happen; instead, if you practice this exercise for five minutes once or twice a day, you will notice that your shoulders and neck will become more flexible and stronger. Be sure to relax your neck and shoulders. The gentle stretch in the wrists helps to prevent repetitive stress injuries from computer work.

3. Gathering the Qi: To Fill Up Your Energetic Gas Tanks

Chinese medicine holds that the body has three main centers or cavities that store energy. These centers are like energetic gas tanks that hold different types of energy for your daily use. The energy center in your head stores spiritual and intellectual energy. The energy center in your chest stores emotional and empathic energy. The energy center in your lower abdomen stores physical energy and is the seat of your overall vitality. This exercise uses visualization to fill all three gas tanks so that you will feel calm, balanced, and revitalized.

1. Stand in *wuji* posture or sit upright in a chair with your feet flat on the floor.

2. Raise your hands to forehead height, with your palms facing your forehead and your elbows either out to the sides or slightly dropped. Your palms should be about a foot away (forward) from your forehead.

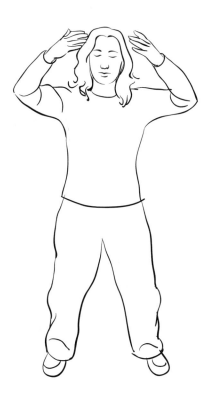

3. Inhale, and visualize sending or pushing qi in the form of white light or white mist into your head, while moving your forearms and hands slightly backward toward your forehead by bending your arms at the elbows.

4. Exhale, pull your hands away to return to the starting position, and visualize a bright light glowing inside your head.

5. Inhale, and push energy into your head like bright white light brightening a dark room.

6. Exhale, and see the bright white light of energy glowing even brighter.

7. Repeat up to 6 times.

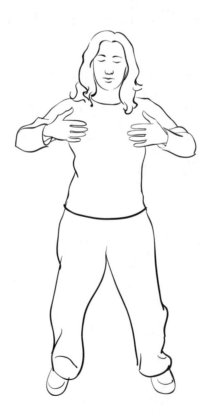

8. Now lower your hands to about a foot in front of your chest with your elbows bowed slightly outward.

9. Inhale, move your hands and forearms toward your chest, and send a calming energy in the form of white light into your chest.

10. Exhale, and pull your arms back about a foot in front of your chest, while visualizing a bright, calming ball of white light inside your chest.

11. Repeat up to 6 times.

12. Lower your hands to face the area just below your belly button. Inhale, and push the qi into your low abdomen.

13. Exhale, and pull your hands to about a foot in front of your belly. See a bright light glowing inside your belly.

14. Repeat up to 6 times.

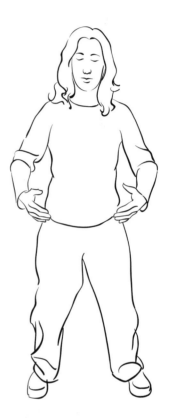

The movements of this exercise are easy: Inhale, and push qi into the energy center as your hands come closer to your body. Exhale, and see a light glowing in the energy center as you bring your hands back to about a foot away from your body. The difficult part of this exercise may occur with your ability to focus your mind on the visualization. Be patient with yourself and don't give up. Over time, this exercise will help you to develop stronger mental focus as it balances the energy throughout your body.

4. Qigong Facial Massage: To Rejuvenate Your Face and Alleviate Tension

Acupressure is a traditional Chinese medicine technique that uses physical pressure to stimulate specific points on the body to relieve and prevent a variety of stress-related ailments. Historically, acupressure evolved from acupuncture; it is based on the same principles of rebalancing vital energy to restore and maintain health.

If you spend a lot of time at the computer, driving, or reading, chances are good that stress is affecting your face. Stress causes facial muscles to become tense, which can lead to unwanted wrinkles and creases over time. There are several acupuncture points on the face that are used to release facial tension; this exercise uses them all. Acupressure facial massage is an excellent wrinkle-preventing, stress-releasing technique to practice when you get into bed or whenever you need some rejuvenation during your day.

1. Stand in *wuji* posture or sit upright in a chair. (You can also do this lying down.)

2. Place the pads of your middle fingers between your eyebrows above your nose.

3. Rub in small circles, in either or both directions; first rub in one direction and then the other.

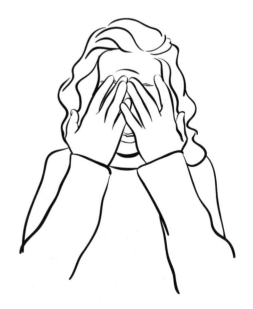

4. Using the pads of your middle fingers, rub with significant pressure along each eyebrow toward your ears. Spend more time on the places that feel the tenderest or the most achy.

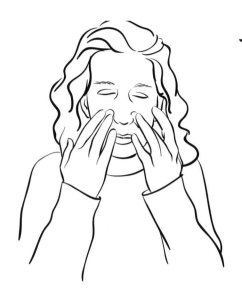

5. Rub your temples and then move your hands and continue to rub under your cheekbones toward your nose. Again, spend more time on places that feel as if they need more attention. Take your time at each spot.

6. Bring your fingers under your ears and a bit forward, to the hinges of your jaw, and rub out any tension that might be there from clenching.

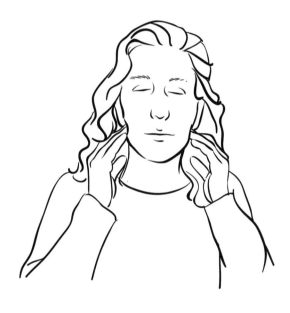

7. Repeat the entire exercise, starting between your eyebrows. Do it as many times as feels good to you.

This whole exercise should take anywhere from two to five minutes. Use these simple acupressure techniques once or twice a day. Pay particular attention to any tender points, which is a sure sign of facial stress. Stimulating your skin this way also will keep it healthier and give it a younger look. I often prescribe this exercise to patients who have jaw pain because of clenching at night; they've reported significant relief in as little as one week of practice.

5. Acupoint Tapping: To Invigorate and Improve Energy Flow

This is one of my favorite exercises to wake me up when I am starting to feel sluggish or when my muscles feel tight. It stimulates areas on the body that are considered *tonifying*, or energizing, to the skin, muscles, internal organs, and brain. It is also the perfect exercise to help disperse aches and blockages that manifest as neck, back, and joint pain.

1. Stand in *wuji* posture or sit upright in a chair.

2. Make a soft fist with one hand. Begin by tapping the area between your neck and your opposite shoulder with the flat part of your fist (where the fingers are curled). You can use a good amount of pressure, but don't hurt yourself.

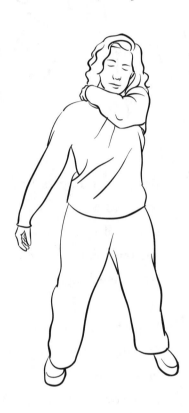

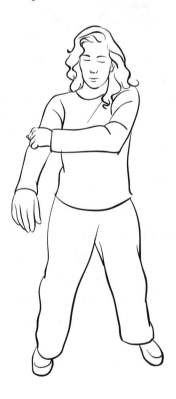

3. Continue to tap slowly down the outside of your arm toward your wrist. Spend more time tapping your fist on those areas that feel tender.

4. When you reach your hand, tap the fleshy area, (sometimes called the heel) between your thumb and first finger; this is a very important point for immunity, headaches, and allergies.

5. Turn over the same arm you've been tapping, and tap down your inner arm from the armpit down toward your wrist.

6. End tapping that side by tapping against the palm of your hand.

7. Switch sides by making a fist with the hand that was just tapped. Then tap the area between your neck and your opposite shoulder.

8. Work your way down the outside of your arm as you did on your other arm.

9. End by tapping the point between your thumb and first finger.

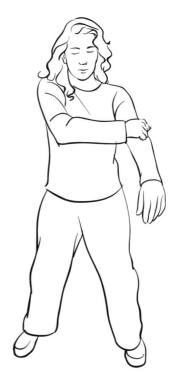

10. Now tap down your inner arm, and end by tapping the palm of your opposite hand.

11. Make two fists and tap your lower back with the backs of both hands. Relax your shoulders. Spend some extra time here and find points in the lower back that feel tight. Tap with a comfortable amount of pressure.

12. Continue tapping down to both sides of your buttocks (left fist at left side, right fist at right side) with the curled-finger part of your fist, and then down the outsides of both legs to your ankles.

13. Come back up and shift tapping your fists to your inner legs; tap down your inner legs to your ankles.

14. End by placing both palms on your abdomen. Smile to yourself and take three deep breaths before ending the exercise.

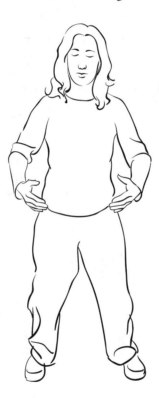

This exercise is a good one to include in the beginning part of a qigong workout. The whole process should take about three to five minutes. It's normal to feel your arms, legs, and back tingling after you finish.

6. Healing Sound for Digestion: To Balance Hunger and Strengthen Your Stomach

From as far back as the Qin Dynasty (221-207 BCE), healing sounds have been used for healing purposes. Healing sound vocalization has an immediate calming effect on your nervous system, which connects with all of your internal organs and tissues. Emphasis is placed on the connections between the area of focus and the mind, breath, and imagination. While you are intoning the therapeutic sound, you should feel enveloped by that sound or vibration.

The healing sound for digestion is *hu* (pronounced "who"). Intoning this sound improves sluggish digestion, helps reduce heartburn, and relieves gas and bloating. It also helps to balance hunger, which can be an important tool when dieting. Chinese medicine views food and drink as two of the three major sources of energy (air is the third). A healthy digestive system ensures good energy levels throughout your day.

1. Stand in *wuji* posture or sit upright in a chair.

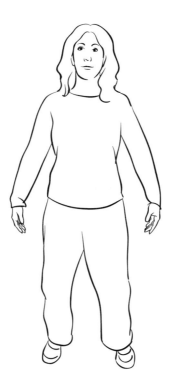

2. Interlace your fingers, raise your hands over your head until your elbows are straight, and twist your hands so that your palms face the sky.

3. Lean slightly to the right to open the area of your body where your spleen and pancreas are located. This will also give your stomach a slight stretch.

4. Inhale and visualize white light filling your stomach.

5. Exhale the *hu* sound as if you were blowing through a straw. You don't need to vocalize the sound; instead, the sound is made by the breath going past your lips. However, you certainly can add your voice to the sound if you wish.

6. As you exhale, visualize hunger, heat, or discomfort being released from your stomach and exiting your body through your mouth with your breath.

7. Repeat 6 to 18 times.

This exercise works wonders with low-grade heartburn and stomachaches, and it can help recalibrate the dynamics of your hunger-fullness cycles. As your digestive system becomes stronger, your body will become more efficient at converting food nutrients into energy.

7. Healing Sound to Blow Off Steam: To Cool Down Your Body

This is one of those exercises that helps you regain your energy when you feel overheated or overwhelmed. When practiced regularly, it helps to prevent headaches and cool down hot flashes. The sound you use is the *she* sound (pronounced like the word "she"). It would be a good idea to review the Cleanse the Qi exercise here, as the breathing is the same, and your hands make the same movements for this exercise as they do in Cleanse the Qi.

1. Begin by standing in *wuji* posture or sitting upright in a chair.

2. On an inhale, raise your arms out to your sides with your palms facing the earth until your arms are at shoulder height. Visualize gathering the calm energy around you as if you were gathering a bright white light.

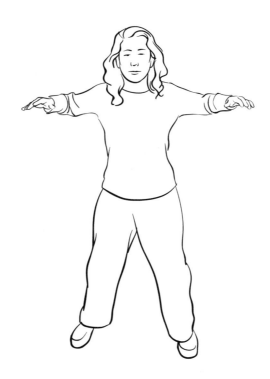

3. While still inhaling, turn your palms up to face the sky and continue to raise your arms over your head. Continue to visualize gathering calm energy around you like a bright white light.

4. Exhale slowly once your arms are almost straight up with your palms facing each other; then slowly bring your hands down the front of your body with your palms facing the earth and your fingertips pointing toward each other. As you exhale, intone the *she* sound either with your voice, or just using the sound of your breath exiting through your mouth.

5. Repeat by inhaling and bringing your arms out to your sides and over your head, then exhaling the *she* sound as you bring your arms down the front of your body with your palms facing the earth.

6. Repeat 6 to 18 times.

When you feel too much heat and pressure from stress, this exercise acts like a pressure valve. Much in the same way that opening a valve releases excess pressure, this exercise frees up the body's energy to circulate more efficiently. I prescribe this exercise regularly for cancer patients undergoing chemotherapy and radiation, which both tend to overheat the body, and for menopausal women suffering from hot flashes.

8. Lung and Breathing Revitalizer: To Increase the Fuel for Your Body's Cells

As mentioned earlier, air, along with food and drink, is considered one of the most powerful ways to boost energy. When I say "air," what I mean is the oxygen content derived from breathing deeply and fully. Most of us can go an entire day (or even many days) without taking a good deep breath. Sitting at a desk limits the lungs' capacity to expand, which is exacerbated by slouching.

This exercise moves your arms to maximize chest expansion, which gives your lungs the room they need to expand more fully. Remember that you are practicing qigong breathing, which means pushing your belly out on the inhale and pulling it back in on the exhale.

1. Place your arms in front of your body at shoulder level, as if you are about to start swimming the breaststroke. Turn your palms down to face the earth. Your elbows should be bent and sticking out from your sides. Your arms should feel as if they are resting on water. Relax your shoulders back and down.

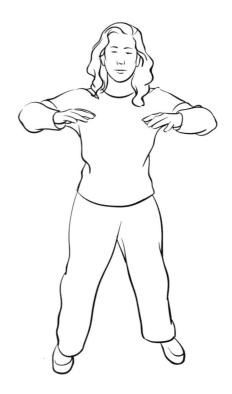

2. Inhale very slowly and bring your arms out to your sides, leading with your elbows. Squeeze your shoulder blades together while keeping your shoulders relaxed.

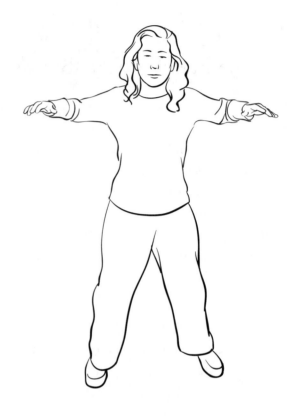

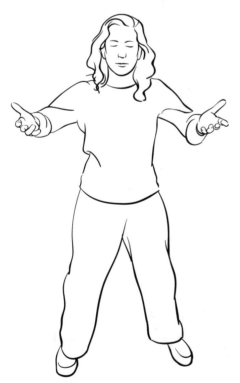

3. Once you can't bring your elbows back any farther, turn your palms up, exhale very slowly, and bring your arms back toward the starting position with your palms up. Keep your arms and hands up at shoulder level in front of your body.

4. As your hands reach the starting position, turn your palms down, inhale, and pull your elbows out to your sides to repeat the exercise.

5. Make sure that your shoulders are relaxed throughout all of the movements.

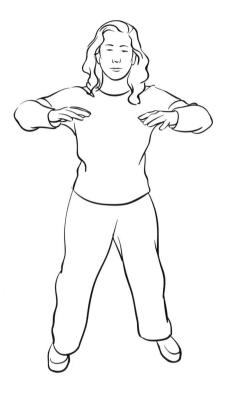

Repeat this exercise for five to ten minutes. The arm movements will help to release tension from your chest, shoulders, and upper back. They will also strengthen your arm muscles over time.

Deep breathing is one of the easiest ways to recharge your body, lower blood pressure, circulate extracellular fluids (lymph), and massage your internal organs. On a chemical level, the more oxygen you provide for your cells, the more fuel they have to function efficiently, making more energy available for use throughout your day.

9. Strengthen Knee Qi: A Boost for Your Knees, Legs, and Feet

As we age, our backs and knees are usually the first parts of our bodies to become chronically sore. However, there is no good reason why we shouldn't be able to continue to exercise, take walks, and ride our bikes when we are seniors. Walking is one of the best ways to get your heart pumping, and it's easy on the body's joints.

This exercise helps ensure that our knees and legs remain strong as we age. There is also a bonus that comes with this exercise, which is the stimulation of the bottoms of both feet. This stimulation provides a mini reflexology massage that stimulates the whole body via the feet.

1. Stand with your feet and knees together. Keep your knees slightly bent.

2. Place both palms on your knees, the left palm on the left knee and the right palm on the right knee. Make sure your neck is in a comfortable position.

3. Rotate your knees together in a circular motion 3 times in a clockwise direction. Make sure that your knees don't stick out past your toes, and allow all of your body's weight to rest on your feet.

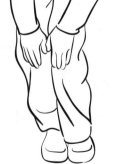

4. Then circle your knees in the opposite direction. Your knees always remain pressed together, and should never come out past your toes.

5. Repeat the circles, 3 in one direction and then 3 in the opposite direction. Pay attention to the sensations on the bottoms of your feet.

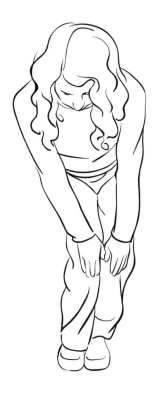

Practice this exercise for a few minutes once or twice a day. This is an ideal warm-up before doing the cardiovascular exercise of your choice. The more you practice, the stronger the quadriceps muscles of your thighs will become, and your leg tendons will become more supple.

10. Strengthen Back Qi: To Release Back Tension

Many of us store stress and tension in our lower backs. Your back can get sore if you spend a large amount of time sitting or standing, and this exercise is the perfect antidote. From a psycho-emotional viewpoint, back pain sometimes manifests when you cannot carry all of the responsibilities or stresses of your daily life. In that instance, your body cries out for relief. This exercise helps to stretch your back to relieve back pain and tension. It feels great, and gives your whole torso a good stretch.

1. Stand with your legs and feet together. Bend your knees slightly and tuck your tailbone under to minimize the curve in your lower back. Place the backs of your hands on your lower back, just below where your rib cage ends.

2. Tilt your whole torso to the left by bending at the waist until you feel a stretch in your right side. Circle your upper body forward and to the right to complete a half circle.

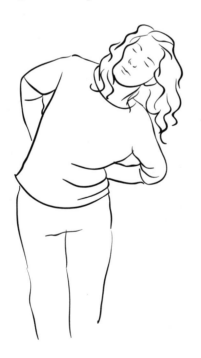
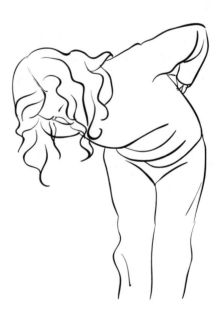

3. When you reach your right side, come back up to a vertical position, and then tilt to the left to circle again for a total of 6 to 9 times. Never lean backward after reaching your right side.

4. Now tilt at your waist to the right, and stretch your left side. Circle forward and around for a total of 6 to 9 times to the left, always coming back to vertical after a half circle rather than tilting backward.

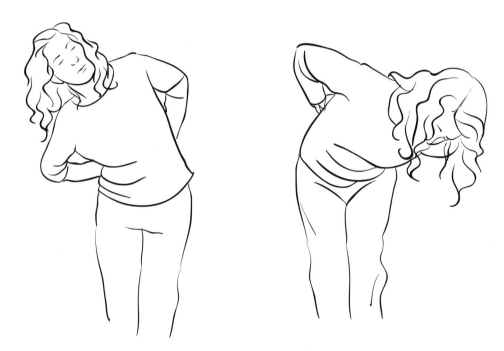

5. Circle in this direction for a total of 6 to 9 times. 🖎

I recommend practicing this exercise immediately before or right after doing the knee exercise (exercise 9), because your legs are already in the correct position. This exercise provides a satisfying stretch for both sides of your lower back. You never tilt your body backward because that movement compresses the spine, which could cause pain or worsen existing pain.

11. Strengthen Wrist Qi: To Avoid Repetitive Stress Injury

We are all spending more and more time on the computer for better or worse. Although a computer makes many aspects of life quicker or easier, it also positions your body in ways that can lead to discomfort and pain if you don't stop frequently to stretch. The following exercise offers two ways to avoid carpal tunnel syndrome and repetitive stress injuries, which are both associated with spending too much time on the computer.

1. Stand in *wuji* posture or sit in an upright position.

2. Place your hands in prayer position, with both palms touching and your fingers pointing toward the sky.

3. Tilt your fingers to face forward as far as you can while keeping your palms pressed together. Get a good stretch in both wrists.

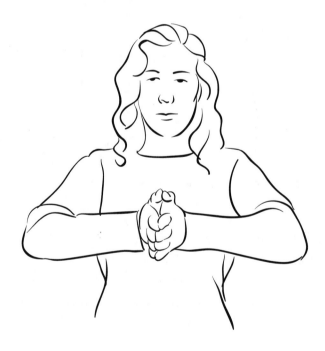

4. From that position, rotate your hands as far as you can so that your fingers point toward your body, again keeping your palms pressed together. Raise your elbows while you do this to get a bigger stretch in the wrists.

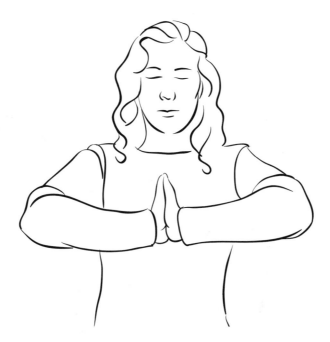

5. Very slowly, alternate the rotation of your hands forward and backward at least 9 times. You can coordinate the movements with each inhale and exhale to make this a meditative exercise. (For example, inhale as your fingers point away, and exhale as your fingers point toward your body.)

6. Now separate your hands and make fists. Hold your fists up at chest level.

7. Roll your fists in circles to stretch your hands and the entire wrist area. Circle at least 9 times.

8. Change the direction of the circles and roll your fists in the opposite direction at least 9 times. Remember to keep your fists at chest level.

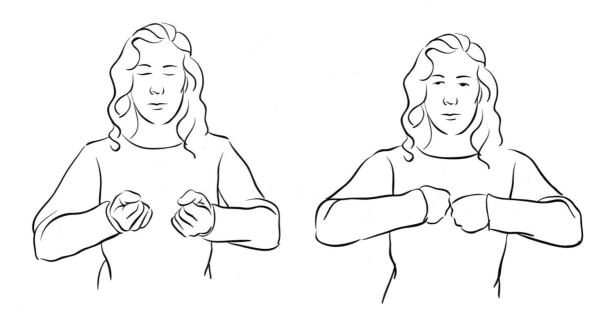

9. To end, shake out both of your hands.

Lately, I've been seeing more and more people who have wrist pain from working on a computer all day. The key to avoiding wrist problems is to stop every hour and practice this exercise. Even if you practice for only two to three minutes, when you do so every hour it really does add up.

12. Neck Qi Flow, Variation I: To Increase Range of Motion

Right now, turn your neck from side to side. Many people can turn more easily or more completely to one side than the other. This can be due to various factors, such as carrying a heavy purse on the same shoulder for years, tension or stress, or perhaps an old injury. The good news is that it's not difficult to regain most—if not all—of your neck's full range of motion. This exercise stretches the neck and the muscles that connect the neck to the shoulders. So with this one, you get two stretches for the price of one: a neck stretch and a shoulder stretch.

1. Stand in *wuji* posture or sit upright in a chair.

2. Push your shoulders back and then down. Be sure to keep them held down throughout this exercise.

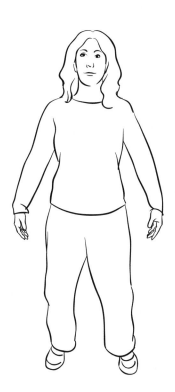

3. Inhale, and turn your head to the left.

4. Exhale, and bring your head back to face forward.

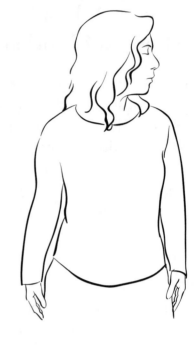

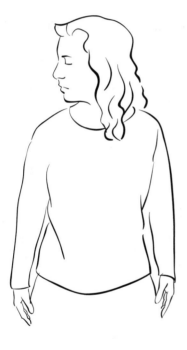

5. Inhale, and turn your head to the right.

6. Exhale, and bring your head back to face forward.

7. Repeat at least 9 times in each direction.

Chronic stress causes the shoulders to move forward and collapse the chest. By holding your shoulders back and down, you are correcting and realigning your posture while releasing tension from your neck and shoulders.

13. Neck Qi Flow, Variation II: To Loosen the Neck and Upper Back

This exercise pairs well with exercise 12. Both exercises help to release stress and tension from the neck and shoulders. This particular exercise has the added benefit of stretching the muscles in the upper back. Tension in the upper back can lead to neck pain and vice versa. This is an easy way to release tension from both areas at the same time.

1. Stand in *wuji* posture or sit upright in a chair.

2. Push your shoulders back and then down. Be sure to keep them held down throughout this exercise.

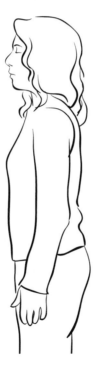

3. Tilt your neck so that your right ear is pointing to or facing your shoulder.

4. Drop your chin and very slowly circle your head down and to the left.

5. Once you reach the left side, bring your neck up to vertical position and then tilt it again so that your right ear points to or faces your right shoulder.

6. Repeat 6 to 9 times.

7. Switch sides, and now tilt your neck so that your left ear points to or faces your left shoulder. Circle very slowly around to the right.

8. When you reach your right side, bring your neck up to vertical position, and then repeat the circular movement from 6 to 9 times.

When practicing this neck roll, try to get a good stretch in your upper back. Pay attention to spots that feel tight as you circle, and breathe into them. To keep this exercise safe and pain free, never tilt your neck back when practicing; you are to make only half circles.

14. Shoulder Qi Flow: To Relax the Shoulders and Open the Chest

When you sit in the same position for too long, or you hold your stress in your neck and upper back, your shoulders usually become tight and stiff. As a result, your shoulders move forward and collapse the chest, leaving little room for a good inhale. This exercise opens the chest and loosens the shoulder joints. When you combine this one with the two neck exercises that precede it, you have the power to improve your upper body posture and range of motion dramatically.

1. Stand in *wuji* posture or sit upright in a chair.

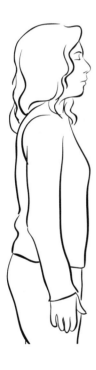

2. Check your posture to make sure that your neck is vertically aligned over your torso (not leaning forward or back).

3. Roll both shoulders in backward circles while inhaling slowly. See if you can inhale for a duration of 3 circles.

4. Exhale slowly, and continue to roll your shoulders in backward circles. See if you can exhale for a duration of 3 circles.

5. Repeat for three to five minutes.

When rolling your shoulders, allow your arms to hang loosely. Try to take big, slow, even breaths to fill your lungs completely. Combining the shoulder rolls and deep breathing helps to relax and stretch the muscles in the front of your neck and chest.

15. Eye Qi Flow: To Relax the Eyes and Strengthen Vision

We use our eyes from the time we wake up until the time we go to sleep. Rarely do we take the time to shut our eyes just to give them a break. Eyestrain and tension can lead to headaches and vision loss. This exercise is one way to give your eyes some relief and energy, which can help to slow down or even prevent the need for glasses, or if you already wear glasses, the need for stronger lenses.

1. First rub your palms together until they're warm.

2. Close your eyes and place your left palm on your left eye and your right palm on your right eye. Inhale, and visualize transferring the heat from your palms to your eyes. "Pull out" the heat from your palms and put it into your eyes. Exhale, and relax your eyes beneath your palms. Continue doing this for up to three breaths, or until the heat has gone from your hands.

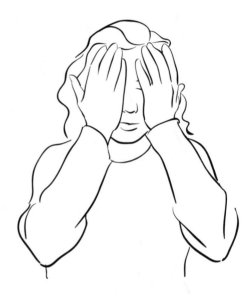

3. With your hands still over your closed eyes, roll your eyes 9 times clockwise and then 9 times counterclockwise.

4. Repeat the entire exercise two more times. 永

Heat is a form of energy, and when you visualize drawing the heat from your palms to your eyes, you are providing your eyes with warm, soothing energy. The heat also relaxes the facial muscles around your eyes. Rolling the eyes strengthens their muscles.

16. Wash Your Face: To Rejuvenate and Revitalize Your Skin

Have you ever splashed water on your face to help yourself wake up? Well, this exercise is kind of like that. Rubbing your hands up and down your face, when coordinated with your breath, energizes your skin while rubbing out tension. I find this exercise comes in handy when I need to finish a task but I don't feel as though I have enough energy to do it. Just a few quick rubs and I am ready to get the job done. Try this for yourself.

1. Stand in *wuji* posture or sit upright in a chair.

2. Place your palms on your face, with your middle fingers level with your nostrils.

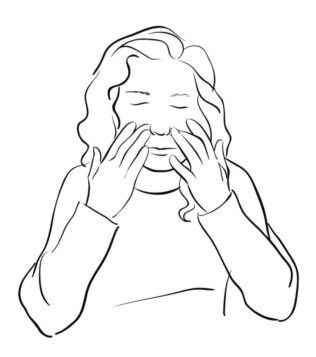

3. Slowly inhale and push your palms against your skin up to your hairline (on your forehead).

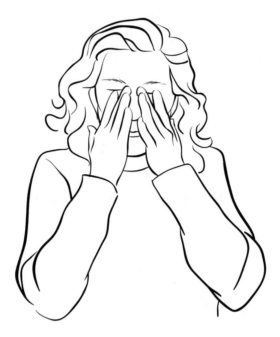

4. Once your palms are on your forehead, exhale quickly and move your hands quickly back down to their starting position, level with your nostrils.

5. Repeat by inhaling and slowly pushing your hands up, and then exhaling quickly as you quickly pull your hands back down, rubbing against your face.

You can do this as many times as you'd like, until you start to feel refreshed. Be sure to breathe only through your nose. This exercise is also great for opening up clogged sinuses, but you'd better have a tissue ready! Try to rub your middle fingers up and down the sides of your nose to enhance the sinus-clearing effects.

17. Qi Scattering: To Bounce Off Old Energy

This one is fun. It makes me feel like a kid when I practice it, because we adults so rarely bounce up and down. Doing it looks a little like professional boxers getting ready for a fight, only without the gloves and the fancy satin shorts. The act of bouncing helps to dispel old stagnant energy from your muscles, sinews, and bones. By bouncing, you can get rid of energy blockages that are slowing you down.

1. Stand in *wuji* posture.

2. Raise your heels off the ground and then lower them back down to the ground in quick succession.

3. Continue to bounce on your heels while keeping your knees, hips, and shoulders loose.

4. Enjoy doing this exercise for as long as you wish to continue it.

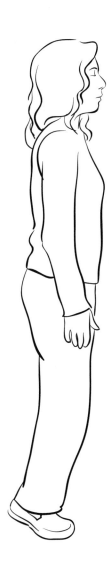

Keep your knees slightly bent to protect your lower back. Allow your arms to bounce freely with your body. This exercise is a great fatigue buster and it really gets your heart going too.

18. Ear Massage: To Invigorate and Balance Your Whole Body

One very popular microsystem of acupuncture uses only the ears to treat the entire body. The history of this treatment is quite interesting. In the 1950s, Paul Nogier, a French medical doctor, discovered that the ear can be seen as a microcosm of the entire body. This means that all the separate parts of the body correspond to separate locations on the ear and, consequently, the ear can be mapped for diagnosis and treatment of the corresponding body part. In 1958, the Chinese government verified his findings, which led to the popularity of ear acupuncture in Chinese medicine clinics in China and abroad. I frequently use ear acupuncture in my clinic, and I can attest to the amazing power it has to balance people's moods and reduce physical pain.

This exercise uses acupressure to stimulate the hundreds of acupuncture points on the ear. There are points that correspond to your internal organs, to specific areas of your brain, to your musculoskeletal system, and to psycho-emotional states.

1. Stand in *wuji* posture, sit in a chair, or lie on your back.

2. Place your thumbs and first fingers on your earlobes. Rub the entire fronts and backs of both earlobes. The earlobes have points that correspond to the parts of your brain that help to balance your mood.

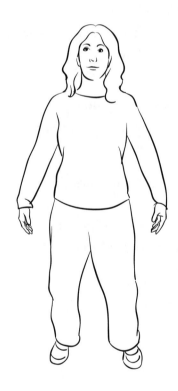

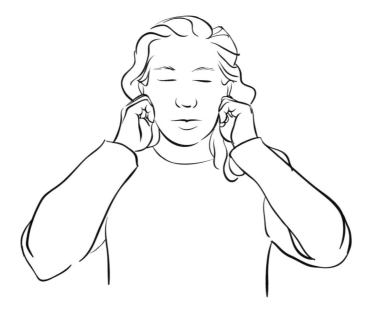

3. Work your way up and around all of your outer ear tissue. Be sure to get the fronts and backs of both ears. These areas correspond to several musculoskeletal points, and they help to relax your back, neck, and limbs.

4. Put your first fingers inside your ears (but not the ear canals), and continue to rub the complete surfaces and all the crevices. This area corresponds to several internal organ points, which help with regulating metabolism and organ function.

5. Once you have rubbed the entire ear, inside and out, go back to rubbing your earlobes to end this exercise.

When you've finished this exercise, your ears should feel hot and tingly. I like to practice this before bed, or when I am feeling moody. It helps to balance the mind and body, and can help you to unwind after a busy day.

19. Gathering Qi in Your Bio-Battery: To Center Your Thoughts

Life has a way of pulling us in many different directions all at once. Our jobs make demands on us, our families have demands, we have scores of responsibilities to attend to, and sometimes it can all get a little overwhelming. A good vacation is the perfect antidote for stress, but sometimes it is hard to get away. This exercise takes you out of your daily responsibilities and helps you feel more grounded and centered. It creates a sense of calm in the midst of a storm.

Your *bio-battery* is located in your lower abdomen. Scientists refer to this as the "digestive brain," and it is one of the three energy centers of the body. Where the mind goes, the qi follows, and focusing on your bio-battery sends energy into your lower abdomen, which creates a feeling of balance from within.

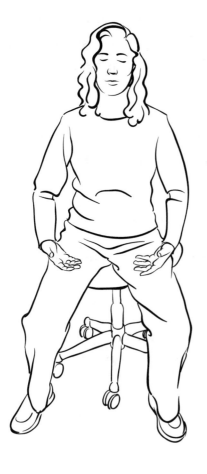

1. Stand in *wuji* posture or sit upright in a chair.

2. Place your palms in front of your abdomen, just below your navel. Have them face, but not touch, your belly. Position your hands as if holding or supporting a big belly.

3. Your elbows remain by your sides so that your wrists do not bend. The position is as if you are holding a big ball.

4. Slightly separate and relax your fingers. Keep your hands about four inches apart, with your fingertips pointing toward each other.

5. When you inhale, visualize your breath filling your belly like a golden mist.

6. When you exhale, see and feel the golden mist in your belly.

7. Continue to hold this position and maintain this visualization for at least five minutes.

8. To end this exercise, feel a state of calm filling your body, originating from your abdomen and continuing upward to your head and arms, downward to your legs and feet, and all the way out to your skin. Let the energy permeate your whole body like steam, until your body is filled all the way out to your skin from within your interior.

Remember to breathe deeply and slowly. Try to keep your mind focused on the visualization. If it starts to wander, bring it back to the image of golden mist filling your abdomen. Over time, this exercise functions like a "mini-oasis," taking you away from your day and bringing you back to yourself. You will feel relaxed, calm, energized, and centered after doing it.

20. Stretching the Spine: To Energize Your Back and Brain

This exercise stretches and aligns your spinal vertebrae while facilitating the flow of energy through your spine all the way up to your head. It stretches the muscles of your whole back, and it feels great. Because it brings fresh blood to the brain, it also helps with mental focus. I often joke with students about doing this exercise right before taking a test. *Caution:* This is for only people who want to loosen up their backs, it is not for people with structural back problems, such as bulging disks, for example. Do not practice this exercise if you have serious back pain. But if you have chronic back and neck tension or soreness, this one's for you.

1. Stand in *wuji* posture.

2. Inhale as you raise both hands above your head, palms facing each other almost like diving into a pool.

3. Exhale and feel your hands getting very heavy. The heaviness pulls your hands forward and down, and then slowly starts to pull the rest of your body over and down beginning with your head. Feel your *cervical vertebrae* (neck bones) stretch as you tilt your head toward the ground. Let the weight of your arms, neck, and head pull on your shoulders, upper back, and middle back. Let that weight pull you forward and down, until you are doing a forward bend with your hands hanging toward the ground. Keep your knees slightly bent the entire time.

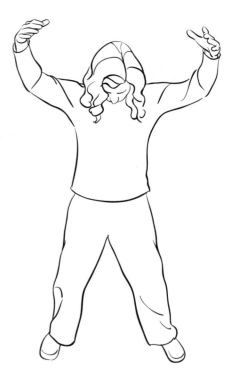

4. Inhale, and rise up by pushing your feet into the ground (keep your knees bent). Let your arms hang as you bring your waist up, then your middle back up, then your upper back up, and then, finally, your neck. Your head is the last part of your body to become vertical.

5. Complete your inhale by raising your hands up into the diving position, before exhaling back down to repeat the exercise.

6. Repeat 6 to 9 times.

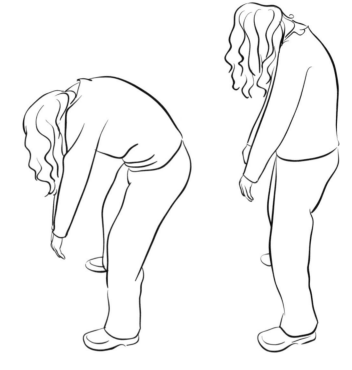

If you encounter pain or any other limitations, honor them and do not push past them. Find your comfort zone and stay within it. The purpose of these movements is to feel each vertebra of the spine stretch sequentially so that a rippling effect descends down the spine when you bend forward, and then back up your spine when you come back to the standing position. When you bend forward, you can visualize stress and tension from your entire body exiting through your arms and flowing out of your hands. When you come back up, you can visualize the energy of the earth slowly filling and energizing your body from your feet up to your head.

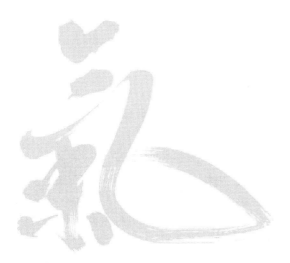

CHAPTER 5

RESTORING
PHYSICAL VITALITY

Many of us come to qigong with health issues that already require attention. That's why this chapter presents exercises that address specific imbalances in the body. Such exercises are called "qigong prescriptions" because they are prescribed (like herbal formulas) to help patients speed their healing. Although there are hundreds of qigong videos that present general exercises for energy, few show you what to do when you don't already have near-perfect health. But clearly, only after you address your own particular health imbalances can you move closer to the goal of optimal vitality.

The best way to use this chapter is to first take an honest look at your physical health. Can your digestion be improved? Do you regularly suffer from low-back pain? How is your sleep? Once you assess the areas that can be improved, look through the exercises in this chapter to find a few that are appropriate for your needs.

This is your chance to empower yourself by taking an active role in your own healing. You will soon realize that a major aspect of healing is an "inside job"; that is, you already possess the innate power to bring yourself closer to a state of good health, whether physical, mental, or spiritual. And even if you are unable to heal your body, you may be able to change how you view your illness. A change of attitude can move you toward a state of greater calm and tranquility.

There is no need to try to practice most or all of the exercises in this chapter. Instead, choose two or three that fit your needs, then practice them diligently. It can take anywhere from a few weeks to a few months to see marked improvement, so be patient. Remember, if you have been suffering from something for a long time, it will take longer to see results.

When you practice these exercises, it is important that you do so mindfully. The more you focus on the exercise while you are practicing, and the more you can keep your mind in the present as you practice, the faster and deeper the results will be. Your body is inherently intelligent, but your consciousness must be focused so that your body will get the message.

As stated earlier, these exercises are not a substitute for medical advice and treatment. If you are currently receiving medical care for a health condition, always check with your doctor before beginning a new exercise routine.

1. Ascend and Descend Earth Qi: To Improve Digestion

Weak digestion is an epidemic in the United States. We've have all seen the amazing number of advertisements and commercials selling drugs for acid reflux, indigestion, constipation, diarrhea, gas, and bloating. Some people say that Americans are overfed and undernourished. Judging from the patients I see in my practice, that saying is absolutely correct. We seem to eat too much of the wrong foods too often, and too little of the foods that our bodies use as fuel to boost our energy and vitality. Over time, these choices weaken our upper digestion (stomach) and lower digestion (intestines), and they leave us feeling heavy, bloated, and fatigued.

When practiced daily, this exercise improves overall digestion; reduces acid reflux, heartburn and nausea; and alleviates constipation. When your digestion has improved, you will be able to extract more energy from your food. Obviously, this exercise will work best if you concurrently commit to changing your eating habits. Today would be a great time to begin increasing the amount of fruits and vegetables you eat every day, and decreasing the amount of greasy and processed foods you consume. How about green tea instead of a soda? A salad instead of fries? Every good choice brings you one step closer to having more energy and feeling great.

This exercise is called Ascend and Descend Earth Qi because in Chinese medicine's Five Element theory, the digestive system fits into the category of earth. (The other four categories are metal, wood, water, and fire.) The color associated with the earth element is yellow, and so you will visualize yellow in the exercise. Also, the human body is seen as a microcosm of the universe, and the "earth" of the body is the abdomen. Therefore, when you see the phrase "earth qi," it means the energy the body uses for digestion.

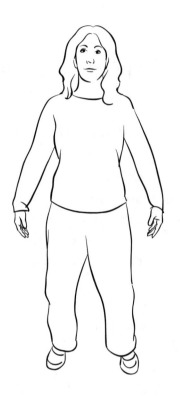

1. Stand in *wuji* posture. Relax every muscle of your body and quiet your mind. Breathe naturally and deeply.

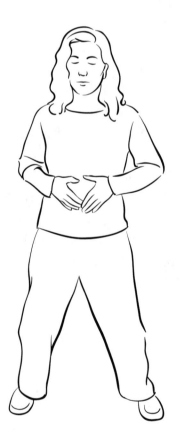

2. Place both palms over your stomach, which is located approximately between the left and right sides of your rib cage, just below your *sternum* (breastbone).

3. Gather the energy of your stomach into each hand, visualizing this stomach energy as two glowing balls of yellow light, one ball in each hand.

4. On an exhale, pull the two balls of qi out to the sides of your torso and down past your waist. (Your left hand pulls down the left side of your body, and your right hand pulls down the right side.)

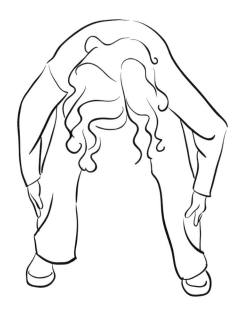

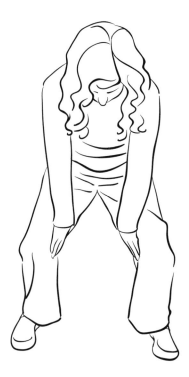

5. During that same exhale, continue to push the balls of yellow qi down the outsides of your legs. Continue by bending lower so that your hands move downward past your outer thighs and knees to your outer ankles. Visualize pushing the qi past your ankles and into the ground.

6. Inhale, shift your palms over your feet to the insides of your ankles, and visualize earth energy gathering from deep in the earth and flowing into your hands.

7. On that same inhale, pull the earth energy up the insides of your legs. Continue pulling the qi up past your inner thighs and into your stomach. Feel the energy fill and energize your stomach.

8. Repeat 18 or 36 times, once or twice a day.

Chances are good that you already know how to improve your eating habits. Why not start now? Chinese medicine places great importance on eating three meals a day, each meal at around the same time each day. Breakfast is the most important meal of the day, and a high-fiber, nutritious breakfast will give you much-needed energy and keep you from being becoming hungrier later in the morning. Never skip breakfast! Also, try to eat dinner at least three hours before bedtime, so that your digestive system can rest when your body is asleep, instead of having to work through the night digesting dinner. Finally, don't wait to eat until you are starving or fatigued. When you wait too long to eat a meal, your food choices are always worse. Bring the mindfulness of your qigong practice to the practice of eating, and you will discover the recipe for success.

2. Heart Qi Massage: To Strengthen Your Heart Function

Much of heart disease is the result of the blockage of blood flow to the heart. This exercise is for those who wish to avoid bypass surgery later in life, or to prevent a second heart surgery if you've already had one. And although this exercise does not reduce high cholesterol, which is also linked to heart disease, it strengthens heart function and blood flow to help counteract the effects of high cholesterol.

If you have high blood pressure or a history of heart disease in your family, this exercise is for you. It is excellent as a preventative measure, but it will also help if you have received a troubling diagnosis from your doctor.

1. Stand in *wuji* posture or sit upright in a chair.

2. Breathe slowly and deeply. Relax your mind and visualize your body melting into the ground with each exhale. Repeat until your whole body feels relaxed.

3. Place one palm on the center of your chest slightly above your breasts, and place your other palm on top of the hand resting on your chest. Try to position your hands so that you can feel your heartbeat under them.

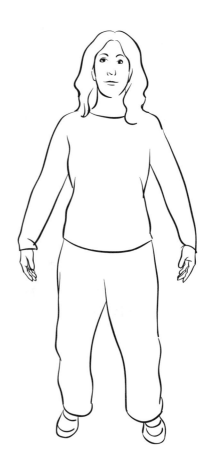

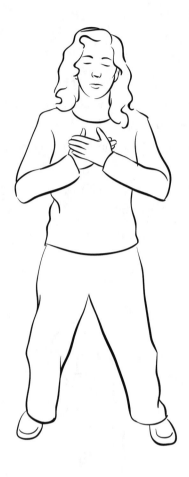

4. Focus your mind on your heart. Visualize massaging your heart while moving your hands in 12 circular rotations clockwise to the left, and then 12 times counterclockwise to the right on the area around your heart.

5. As you circle clockwise and counterclockwise, focus your mind's intention on your heart, visualizing the energy of your heart circulating and flowing in accord with the movement of your hands, as if your hands were magnets.

6. After circling, bring your hands back to the starting position resting over your heart. Concentrate on your heart and try to visualize it in your mind's eye.

7. As you inhale (always through your nose), visualize the breath entering and energizing your heart like a white mist while, at the same time, you lift your hands about one or two inches away from your chest.

8. Exhale (always through your nose) while lightly pressing your chest with your hands, imagining energy glowing like a vibrant red light coming out of your heart as you press.

9. Inhale, and lift your hands about an inch or two away from your heart as you visualize white energy flowing like mist into your heart.

10. Exhale and feel your heart glowing with bright red light as you press your hands on your chest.

11. Repeat for 18 to 36 breath cycles.

12. Close the exercise by visualizing the energy in your heart flowing down and melting into your belly on your final exhale.

The rotating action around the heart promotes blood circulation and disperses *blood stasis* (a situation in which the blood is not circulating optimally through the coronary arteries and heart). Visualizing white energy going into the heart and red energy glowing from out of the heart cleanses *turbid* qi (old or stagnant qi) from the heart, strengthens heart function, and promotes blood flow. When you finish the exercise, your mind and mood should feel relaxed and balanced.

3. Liver Qi Massage: To Detoxify Your Body and Your Moods

No matter who you are, it's likely that your liver could use some TLC (tender loving care). The liver is responsible for detoxifying the pollutants that enter your body via air, food, and drink. Unfortunately, we are exposed to more pollutants today than ever before in history, and it is the liver that bears the brunt of dealing with these toxins. The liver filters the blood and produces the bile necessary for digestion. Furthermore, it helps to regulate both hormones and blood sugar, making it the body's largest gland. All in all, the liver performs hundreds of essential functions.

From the point of view of Chinese medicine, the liver is the organ connected to stress, anger, irritability, and depression. If you suffer from any of these on a chronic basis, Chinese medicine would say that the flow of your liver qi has become stagnant and blocked, which then prevents you from easily returning to a good mood. This in turn impedes the liver's physiological functions and, over time, can weaken this essential organ.

The good news is that the liver is quite able to regenerate itself when given the opportunity. If you have a history of heavy alcohol drinking or working with chemicals, this next exercise will help your liver to detoxify your blood and body.

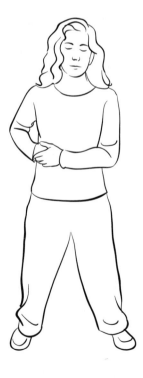

1. Stand in *wuji* posture or sit upright in a chair.

2. Breathe slowly and deeply. Relax your mind and visualize your body melting into the ground on each exhale. Repeat until your whole body feels relaxed.

3. Place one palm on the lower part of your right rib cage, toward the right side of your body. This is where your liver is located. Place your other hand on top of the hand on your rib cage.

4. Focus your mind on your liver, and visualize massaging it while moving your hands in 12 circular rotations clockwise to the left. Then do 12 circular rotations counterclockwise on the lower part of your right rib cage.

5. As you circle clockwise and counterclockwise, focus your mind's intention on your liver, visualizing the energy of the liver circulating and flowing along with the movement of your hands, as if your hands were magnets.

6. After circling, place your hands back to the starting position over your liver. Concentrate on your liver and try to visualize it in your mind's eye.

7. As you inhale (always through the nose), visualize the breath entering and energizing your liver like a white mist, while lifting your hands about one or two inches away from your body.

8. Exhale (always through your nose) while lightly pressing your right rib cage with your hands. Imagine your liver emitting a glowing green energy like a vibrant green light as you press.

9. Inhale and lift your hands about an inch or two away from your liver as you visualize white energy flowing into your liver.

10. Exhale and feel your liver glowing with bright green light as you press your hands on your right rib cage below your chest.

11. Repeat for 18 to 36 breath cycles.

12. Close this exercise by visualizing the energy in your liver melting down into your belly to fill your whole abdomen on your final exhale.

The practice of breathing slowly and deeply during this exercise relaxes the nerves, which in turn has a relaxing effect on the liver. Similarly, according to Chinese Five Element theory, the color green is used to target and strengthen the liver. Over time, you may notice that you have become less irritable or that your depression has started to lift. This is an indication that your liver function is improving, and that the liver qi is flowing freely and smoothly, as it should.

4. Stomach Qi Massage: To Aid and Improve Digestion

As discussed earlier in this chapter, poor digestion is an epidemic in this country, so if it's any comfort, you are not alone. We are encouraged to eat whatever is most convenient, as quickly and cheaply as possible. But the digestive system can sustain this type of lifestyle for only so long before crying out for some help. The cry often takes the form of acid reflux, heartburn, gas, and bloating.

1. Stand in *wuji* posture or sit upright in a chair.

2. Breathe slowly and deeply. Relax your mind and visualize your body melting into the ground with each exhale. Repeat until your whole body feels relaxed.

3. Place one palm over your stomach, between the left and right sides of your rib cage, just below your *sternum* (breastbone). This is the approximate location of your stomach. Place your other hand on top of the hand on your stomach.

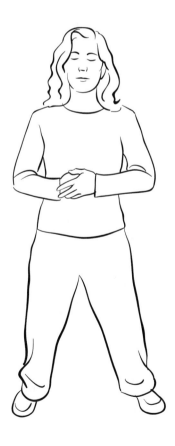

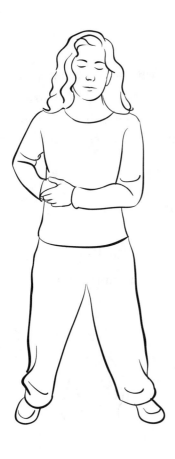

4. Focus your mind on your stomach, and visualize massaging it while moving your hands on your stomach area in 12 circular rotations clockwise to the left, and then 12 times counterclockwise to the right.

5. As you circle clockwise and counterclockwise, focus your mind's intention on your stomach, visualizing the energy of the stomach circulating and flowing along with the movement of your hands, as if your hands were magnets.

6. After circling, place your hands back to the starting position over your stomach. Concentrate on your stomach and try to visualize it in your mind's eye.

7. As you inhale (always through the nose), visualize the breath entering and energizing your stomach like a white mist while, at the same time, lifting your hands about one or two inches away from your body.

8. Exhale (always through the nose) while lightly pressing your stomach with your hands, imagining energy glowing like vibrant yellow light coming out of your stomach as you press.

9. Inhale and lift your hands about an inch or two away from your stomach as you visualize white energy flowing into it.

10. Exhale and feel your stomach glowing with bright yellow light as you press your hands on your stomach.

11. Repeat for 18 to 36 breath cycles.

12. Close the exercise by visualizing the energy in your stomach melting down into your belly on your final exhale.

One easy way to improve your digestion is to chew your food thoroughly. Remember, your stomach doesn't have teeth! If you don't chew well, the larger food particles remain undigested and can accumulate harmful bacteria, which then causes gas and bloating. Digestion begins in the mouth with your saliva, so give your saliva a chance to do its job by chewing your food thoroughly before swallowing.

Finally, slow down when you eat. Sit and eat mindfully. This allows you to know and feel when you have had enough and are full—before you eat too much and become bloated. This also encourages the nerves of your digestive system to relax, and that powerfully aids digestion. Note that you have more nerves in your digestive system than anywhere else in your body.

5. Lung Qi Massage: To Improve Your Respiration and Immunity

Our lungs are usually the first organ to suffer when we get sick. The throat, which is the pathway to the lungs, becomes sore, and the lungs become congested, phlegmy, and inflamed. I've also noticed that both the common cold and flu have become stronger over the years, often leaving people with coughs that last for weeks and weeks. This exercise helps restore strength to the lungs, so the chances of catching a cold or the flu diminish.

If you suffer from allergies or asthma, this is the exercise for you! I used to suffer from severe allergenic and exercise-induced asthma and chronic respiratory infections, so I know what it's like to be unable to take a good breath. It took me years of effort, but I no longer suffer from asthma, and I am rarely sick. How did I do it? I switched to a healthier diet, began exercising moderately, and practiced qigong exercises like this one, which helps strengthen the lungs and the immune system. I'm speaking from experience when I say that this exercise is exceptionally beneficial.

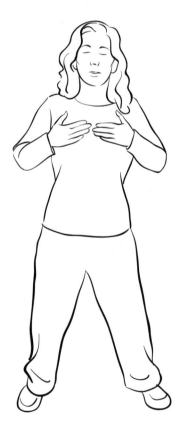

1. Stand in *wuji* posture or sit upright in a chair.

2. Breathe slowly and deeply. Relax your mind and visualize your body melting into the ground on each exhale. Repeat until your whole body feels relaxed.

3. Place your left palm on the left side of your chest, and your right palm on the right side of your chest, with both hands lower than your collarbones. Your lungs are safely housed within your rib cage.

4. Focus your mind on your lungs, and then circle both hands out, down along the outsides of your breasts, in toward your midline, and back up the midline between your breasts to the starting position. (The midline is an imaginary line running down the front of your body from the top of your head, between your eyes, down between your breasts, over the navel, and down to the groin.) Rotate your hands in this manner 12 times, and then switch to 12 times in the opposite direction, which means bringing the hands down between your breasts, out to the sides, and then back up to the chest around and above your breasts.

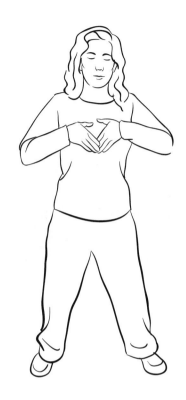

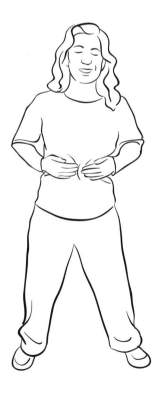

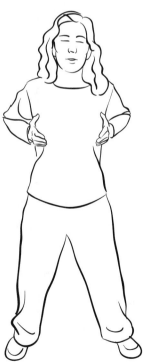

5. As you circle around your lungs, focus your mind's intention on your lungs beneath your hands, visualizing the energy of the lungs circulating and flowing along with the movement of your hands, as if your hands were magnets.

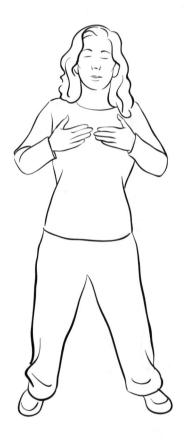

6. After circling, place your hands back in the starting position; that is, with your hands on your chest. Concentrate on your lungs and try to visualize them

7. As you inhale (always through the nose), visualize the breath entering and energizing your lungs like a white mist while, at the same time, lifting your hands about one or two inches away from your body. Visualize the energy filling your lungs from their bottoms to their tops.

8. Exhale (always through the nose) while lightly pressing your chest with your hands. Imagine energy glowing like vibrant white light coming out of your lungs as you press.

9. Inhale and lift your hands about an inch or two away from your lungs as you visualize white energy flowing like mist into your lungs.

10. Exhale and feel your lungs glowing with bright white light as you press your hands on your chest.

11. Repeat for 18 to 36 breath cycles.

12. Close the exercise by visualizing the energy in your lungs melting down into your belly on your final exhale.

Because oxygen is a form of fuel for your cells, the deeper you inhale, the more energy you will have. This energy will help keep your immune system strong, and you may notice that you catch colds less often, or perhaps you will notice that your allergies have lessened. Either way, your lungs will feel stronger, and you will be able to breathe in more vitality and energy.

6. Low-Back and Kidney Massage: To Relax the Muscles of Your Back

Who hasn't suffered from low-back pain at some point in their life? The low back can hurt because of a structural issue, such as an injury or a bulging disk, but it can also be weak and sore due to stress and burn-out. Sitting in one position for too long without stretching, as well as pushing too hard at the gym, can also lead to chronic low-back pain.

The low back houses the kidneys, which in Chinese medicine are the organs responsible for how quickly or slowly we age. It is said that if you push too hard or live in a state of chronic stress, you drain your kidney qi, which leads to premature aging as well as to low-back pain and generalized body aches and pains. This exercise helps to remove tension from the muscles of the low back; it also gives the kidneys an energy boost to help prevent low-back weakness and ache, which are common signs of aging.

1. Stand in *wuji* posture or sit upright in a chair. (I recommend standing if you can.)

2. Breathe slowly and deeply. Relax your mind and visualize your body melting into the ground on each exhale. Repeat until your whole body feels relaxed.

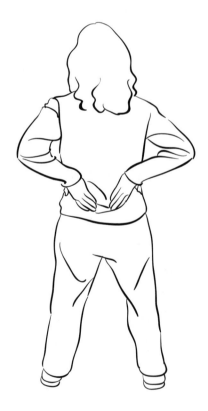

3. Place both palms on your low back below the your rib cage. Focus your mind on your kidneys, which are beneath your lower ribs. Vigorously rub both hands on your low back; first toward the spine and then away from the spine to create warmth and heat in your low-back area. Repeat 36 to 54 times, or until you begin to get tired.

4. After rubbing your low back until it is warm, bring your hands back to the starting position by placing both hands on your low back. Concentrate on your kidneys and try to visualize them in your mind's eye.

5. As you inhale (always through the nose), visualize the breath entering and energizing your kidneys like a white mist while, at the same time, lifting your hands about one or two inches away from your body.

6. Exhale (always through the nose) while lightly pressing your back with your hands, imagining energy glowing like a vibrant dark blue light coming out of your kidneys as you press.

7. Inhale and lift your hands about an inch or two away from your back as you visualize white energy flowing like mist into your kidneys.

8. Exhale and feel your kidneys glowing with dark blue light as you press your hands on your low back.

9. Repeat for 18 to 36 breath cycles.

10. Close the exercise by visualizing the energy in your kidneys moving forward and melting into your belly on your final exhale.

This is a great exercise to bring direct awareness to an area of your body that is likely to be tense or sore. The blue light is said to calm, cool, and soothe the nerves of the low back while energizing the kidneys. You turn your hands into heating pads to soothe and relax your low-back muscles, while giving your bio-battery a much-needed boost.

7. Standing Tree Meditation: To Increase Strength and Combat Fatigue

This ancient meditative qigong exercise simultaneously trains the mind, strengthens the internal organs, and calms the nervous system. It dramatically strengthens the upper and lower body and provides a sense of personal power, which arises from a disciplined meditative practice.

I often tell my students that this is the most powerful way to build strength and energy; even more powerful than the exercises involving movement. One student came to me after practicing this exercise for two months; she said she had lost twenty pounds. She had changed nothing else in her daily routine other than practicing this exercise!

You will use your own body's weight as resistance, so this exercise can be seen as a form of weight training, or as a weight-bearing exercise, which helps keep your bones strong as you age. We all lose muscle mass as we get older, but if you practice this exercise regularly, your legs and arms will remain strong, and you will amass large quantities of qi for use throughout your day.

Do not be discouraged if you find it hard to hold this posture. This is called a meditation practice because we all must practice until we have mastered the meditation postures.

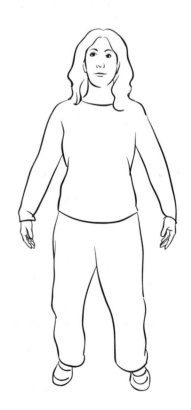

1. Stand in *wuji* posture. Breathe slowly and deeply, using abdominal breathing throughout the exercise. Stand with your weight on all four corners of your feet, which means that your big toe, your pinky toe, and both sides of your heels have your weight distributed equally on them. Take the time to find a comfortable stance, as you will not be moving your legs during this practice.

2. Raise your arms up in front of your chest as if you are hugging a big ball held between your arms and chest.

3. Relax your fingers with your fingertips pointing toward the opposite hand. Your hands should be slightly lower than your shoulders and your thumbs should be relaxed.

4. Place your wrists about your shoulders' distance apart, and place your elbows slightly lower than your wrists.

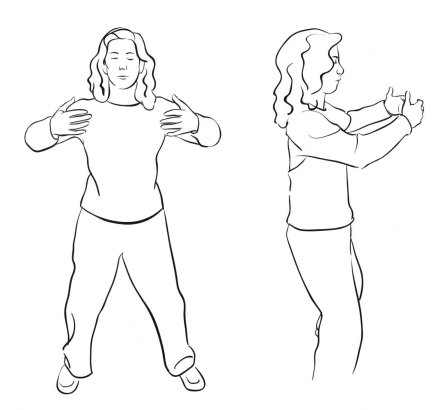

5. Bend your elbows so that the angle between the upper and lower arms is wider than 90 degrees.

6. Continue to breathe deeply and slowly, inhaling as your abdomen expands, and exhaling as your abdomen contracts.

7. Visualize that you are gently holding a large inflated ball between your arms and chest. You are holding this ball in place with no tension whatsoever.

8. If your arms become heavy, visualize them floating or bobbing on water as they hold the ball.

9. Allow the weight of your arms to flow down your back by relaxing the your shoulders back and down. Periodically, check your shoulders to make sure that they are relaxed.

10. Hold this posture for five minutes. Work your way up to five minutes if it is too hard to start there. The ultimate goal is ten to fifteen minutes, once a day.

That is the entire exercise. Below are two suggestions to help you hold the posture longer:

1. Bring your attention to your feet. Visualize tree roots sprouting out of the bottoms of your feet and pushing down deep into the earth. With each inhale, visualize pulling the energy of the earth into your roots, up your legs, and into your lower abdomen.

2. You can also visualize a bright golden thread holding your whole body upright like a puppet. The thread is emerging from the crown of your head and connecting you to the energy of the sky.

It is perfectly normal to feel tension, aches, or muscle fatigue while practicing this exercise. It is deceptively simple but extremely powerful, as it trains the body to accumulate and store large amounts of energy once you've moved past the initial limitations of your muscles.

This standing meditation posture enhances the flow of energy from the bottoms of the feet to the upper body. It strengthens the muscles of the arms, shoulders, and neck. It can take weeks or even months to be able to stand like this comfortably for five minutes a day, but when you feel the energy boost from this practice, the wait will have been worth it.

8, Healing Sound: For High Blood Pressure

Sound vocalization, which penetrates all of your internal organs and tissues, has a directly calming effect on your nervous system. Emphasis is placed on the connection of mind, breath, and imagination to the area of focus. Sound vibrates through the body's internal cavities between the bones and within the organs, and that vibration helps to release stuck qi and tension.

High blood pressure is caused by many factors, including lifestyle and genetics. If you have high blood pressure in your family history, start a preventive routine now. Change to a healthier diet, get better sleep, practice stress-reduction techniques (like qigong), and take naps when you can. All of these activities have been shown to have a positive effect on cardiovascular health.

Jung is the healing sound for high blood pressure (hypertension). *Jung* is pronounced so that it rhymes with "young." You will use this sound in conjunction with a powerful waterfall visualization to enhance the effects of the exercise.

1, Stand in *wuji* posture or sit upright in a chair with the backs of your hands resting on your thighs. Hold your elbows slightly out so that the your armpits are open.

2, Inhale a deep relaxed breath into your lower abdomen. Imagine that you are standing or sitting underneath a beautiful waterfall.

3, Exhale and imagine the feeling of warm water being gently poured over your head, while you make the *jung* sound using either a whisper or by sounding your voice.

4, As you exhale the *jung* sound, feel the water flow down the front, back, and sides of your body, taking with it all tension and heat. Visualize your body being coated with and bathed by the water until the water reaches your feet and saturates the ground around you.

5. Inhale into your lower abdomen, and then exhale the *jung* sound while visualizing warm water flowing down your body as it takes all the heat and tension out from your body and through the bottoms of your feet.

6. Repeat this cycle 18 to 36 times, once a day (twice a day if you have been diagnosed with high blood pressure).

7. End by focusing your attention on the bottoms of your feet. Visualize inhaling into and exhaling out of your feet for a minute or two.

People with high blood pressure often breathe only into the upper areas of their lungs. On the inhale, their shoulders and upper chest will rise, but the remainder of their body is still. Breathing in this way causes an accumulation of qi and tension in the upper body, particularly around the heart and neck.

Abdominal breathing, which is the breathing technique used throughout this book, is how we all breathed before we consciously experienced stress in our lives. It drops the qi from the upper body into the lower body, and will lower blood pressure while performed. Therefore, if you do nothing more than practice slow, deep abdominal breathing for five to ten minutes, twice a day, you will have a blood-pressure-lowering effect on your body.

9. Kneading Your Nose: To Open Your Sinuses

These days, it seems as if every season is allergy season. Sniffling, sneezing, and sinus pain are occurring year-round. Many people suffer from sinus headaches and chronic facial pain due to congested sinuses. This exercise is like a qigong antihistamine, because it helps the sinuses to open.

1. Sit comfortably in a chair.

2. Rub the outsides of your thumbs together until they become warm or hot.

3. Place the outsides of your thumbs on both sides of your nose.

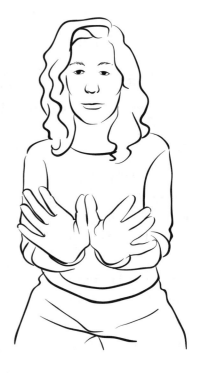

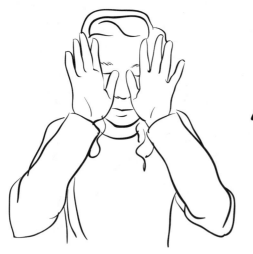

4. Slowly but vigorously rub up and down the sides of your nose using the entire side of each thumb for about 10 breaths. Rub up to your eyes and down to your nostrils.

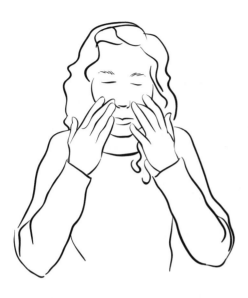

5. Place the tips of your middle fingers on either side of your nostrils; that is, in the depressions to the sides of the nostrils.

6. Rub in small circles, using strong pressure.

7. Continue this rubbing method laterally—out to and across your cheeks—until your fingers are directly below your eyes and aligned under the pupils of your eyes.

8. Slowly work your way back across your cheeks to your nose, and then rub up along the sides of your nose to your eyes.

9. Bring your middle fingers to the place where your eyebrows begin, right above your nose, and rub in small circles for a few breaths.

10. Repeat the entire exercise 9 to 18 times.

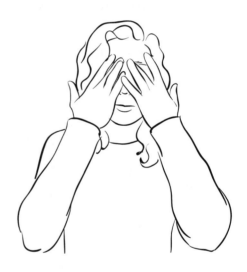

One added benefit of this exercise is that it relieves tension in the facial muscles. By rubbing away facial tension, you can slow down the aging effects of stress on the face. It also leaves you with a glowing complexion. I recommend that you start practicing this exercise a few months before your allergies normally appear.

10. Ten Dragons Run Through the Forest: For Headaches

It is well-known that stress can lead to headaches. Headaches also can occur when you catch a cold or flu, or from using your eyes too much. Neck tension can also lead to headaches. This exercise stimulates the flow of energy through the acupuncture *meridians* (channels) that run along the sides of the head and along the neck to the shoulders. Pain and tension are both dispersed when the qi flows smoothly through these meridians.

There is a saying in Chinese medicine that states, "Where there is blockage, there is pain." This exercise helps move the blockages in the head that lead to headaches. The ten dragons here are your ten fingers. The forest is your head hair. Don't worry, even if you no longer have your hair. It still works!

1. Place all ten of your fingertips at the front of your hairline above your eyes, with your left hand to the left of your hairline's midline, and your right hand to the right of the midline.

2. Point your fingertips toward the back of your head.

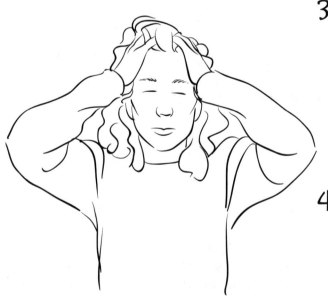

3. Rub all ten fingers along your scalp, from your hairline in front to all over your head and down to your neck. Your fingers act like rakes, so keep them comfortably spread apart.

4. Visualize your hands gathering energy from out of your head and neck as your fingers continue to rake down to your shoulders.

5. Once your hands reach your shoulders, visualize gathering the qi energy in each hand and then toss it down into the earth.

6. Once you have the motion, try to inhale as your hands move from your head to your shoulders, and exhale when you toss the gathered qi.

7. Repeat 18 to 36 times.

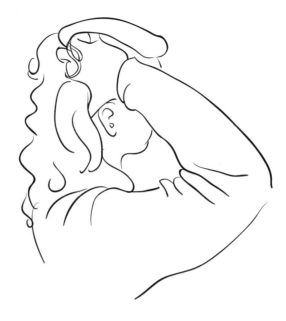

This exercise also can be used to revitalize your mind after you've been focusing on something for too long. It stimulates the skin and the hair on your head, and has an immediate cooling-down effect. It can be wonderfully refreshing at the end of a long day.

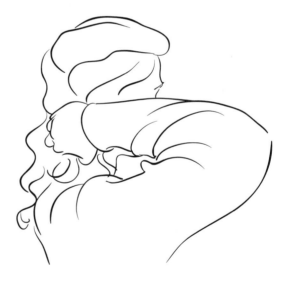

11. Winding the Belt Channel: For Back Pain or Period Pain

I often counsel those who sit at work all day to take breaks every hour and do some gentle stretching. If you sit for long hours on your job, this is the exercise for you. This helps prevent muscle tension and soreness; it also gets your energy and blood flowing to invigorate your body and mind. The *belt channel* is the acupuncture meridian that circles your torso like a belt. When you sit too long in the same position, the energy of that channel becomes stagnant, which leads to pain or soreness in your low back and waist.

This exercise is also effective for menstrual cramps and associated back pain. You should begin practicing this the day or even the week *before* you normally experience back pain or cramps. Note that it may take up to three months before you'll see significant improvement, but be assured that you are loosening the muscles of your back and abdomen in this process, and that alone makes this exercise worth practicing.

If you have (or had) a back injury, check with your doctor before you start practicing this one. It's fine if your back feels a little tight or sore while doing this exercise, but if there is any pain, you should stop immediately. Try to do it again more slowly and with more control. If the pain still persists, then you should not practice this exercise. Perhaps you can try gentle stretches toward touching your toes, for a month or so and then try this again.

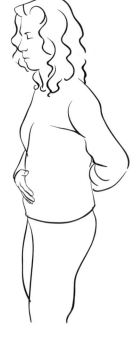

1. Stand in *wuji* posture.

2. Place the back of your left hand on your low back against your spine, and put your right palm on your navel.

3. Turn to the left from your waist to get a nice twist in the waist (keep your knees facing forward), and then circle your upper body toward the right, with your arms out in front of you, and with your palms facing the ground at waist height. Your hands come around with your torso, as if skimming the top of a lake.

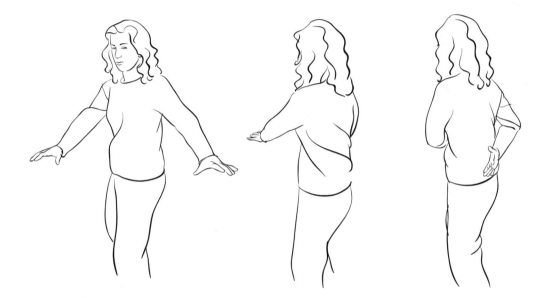

4. When your upper body reaches your right side, let your hands softly hit your body around your waist area.

5. Bring your hands back to the starting position with your left hand on your low back and your right hand on your navel.

6. Turn from your waist to the left and repeat the circle 9 to 18 times.

7. If you can, inhale while you are twisting, and exhale as you bring your hands back to the starting position.

8. Now place your right hand on your low back and your left hand on your navel. Turn from the waist to the right to get a good stretch, while keeping your knees facing forward. Circle to the left with your hands out in front of you, palms facing the earth at waist height.

9. Let your hands gently hit your body when you finish the turn, and then bring them back to starting position before twisting again. Repeat the circle 9 to 18 times.

10. To end, place both hands on your navel, one hand on top of the other, and take three slow, deep breaths.

The twisting movement should be a controlled gentle twist to your back. This twist squeezes your internal organs, giving them a massage. It also stimulates *peristalsis*, which is the movement of food through your digestive tract. I recommend getting up from your chair and practicing this exercise every hour. It will help with your low back, even if you do it for only three minutes each time you do it.

12. Acupoint Stimulation: For Headaches

Acupoint stimulation uses acupressure techniques on specific acupuncture points to elicit a therapeutic response from your body. These points are often needled during an acupuncture treatment, but you have the ability to stimulate these points without needles and without ever having to leave your home! Here is a simple acupoint prescription for headaches.

1. Sit upright in a chair.

2. Rub the fleshy area between your thumb and first finger. Use the thumb and first finger of the opposite hand to squeeze with pressure while you rub. Find the most tender area and continue squeezing and rubbing that area for a few minutes. Then switch hands and rub the same point on your opposite hand using the same technique. (This is the first acupressure point.)

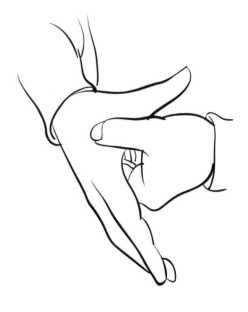

3. Now follow the space on your hand between the knuckles of your ring and pinky fingers down between the bones of your hand. The targeted area is between your knuckles and your wrist, but much closer to the knuckles. It lies between the bones and is sensitive when pressed. Rub that area with your thumb for a minute or two, and then switch to the same point on the opposite hand.

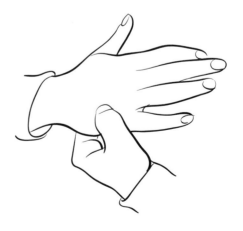

4. If these first two points did not lessen your headache, you can add this third point. Try rubbing the back of the neck where your neck meets your head. There are indentations on either side of the neck vertebrae, and they will be tender. Rub with pressure in circles for a few minutes, and then end by rubbing down your neck toward your shoulders.

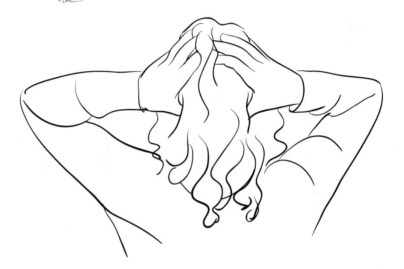

It is important to breathe slowly and deeply while you stimulate all three of these points. Sometimes it's helpful to visualize the pain from your head moving down into the acupoints as you are rubbing them. If you get headaches on a regular basis, you can also use this point prescription to prevent headaches from coming on by stimulating the three points once a day for several weeks.

13. Acupoint Stimulation: For Nausea

Many positive studies have been reported on the benefit of acupuncture and acupressure for nausea, and the *sea bands* (wristbands that stimulate an acupuncture point near your wrist) that you find in drugstores are a direct result of these studies (Lee and Done 1999). Here is a simple acupoint prescription using the "seasickness" acupoint, which has become so famous for treating nausea.

1. Sit upright in a chair.

2. Hold up three fingers with your right hand. Rest the entire outside of your ring finger against and along the left wrist crease on the inside of your left arm. You will also be resting the pads of your three fingers on your forearm. The acupoint is located between the two tendons in the middle of your forearm, where the outside of your first finger meets your forearm.

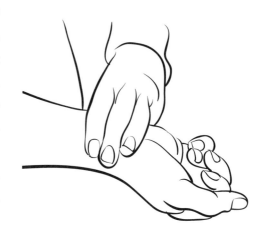

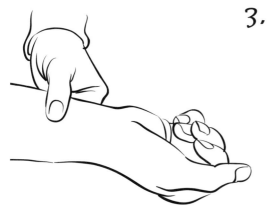

3. Once you've found the point, place your right thumb on it and remove the other fingers of your right hand. Use your right thumb to rub in circles with pressure on the point. You can also squeeze and hold this point for a few minutes, and then repeat the process for another few minutes, if necessary.

4. Switch hands and find the same point on the your right forearm. Squeeze and hold the point, and rub the point in circles using good pressure.

5. To end, focus on your breath. Inhale into your belly, and with each exhale, visualize the energy of your body moving down, starting from your face, past your stomach, down your legs, and then out through your feet. Continue to breathe in this manner, focusing on the downward movement of each exhale for 18 breaths. 祀

There are many causes of nausea. If you have food poisoning, vomiting is an effective way to rid your body of the culprit, and you shouldn't try to prevent it. However, this exercise can still help with the nausea before and even after vomiting. Sometimes people become nauseated when they are nervous or emotionally agitated. This is a great acupoint for such occurrences, as it helps to calm your mind and nerves while calming your stomach.

14, Acupoint Stimulation: For Anxiety

We all experience anxiety on occasion. For example, when you are running late for work, or you can't find your keys or wallet, or you are in an awkward social situation, anxiety makes its appearance. Anxiety and nervousness both have an upward-moving quality, like the feeling of "butterflies" in your stomach that moves up to your head. Deep breathing into and out of your abdomen is one easy way to calm your nervous system. This acupoint prescription is another anxiety-combating tool.

1, Sit upright in a chair.

2, Find the *crown point* of your head. It's at the highest point of your head (the top of the skull). If you place your index fingers on the tops of your ears and go directly up along your head until your fingers meet, you'll find your crown point.

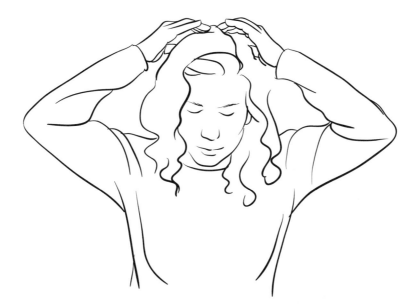

3, Use the first and middle fingers of one hand to press down on your crown point. Breathe slowly and deeply.

4. As you press down, visualize any anxiety or nervousness being forced down your body and out from your feet with each exhale.

5. You can continue to press, or you can also tap on the point. Experiment to see which has the stronger effect for you.

6. Stimulate your crown point for a minute or two.

7. Now take a middle finger and press on your third-eye point, located exactly between your two eyebrows.

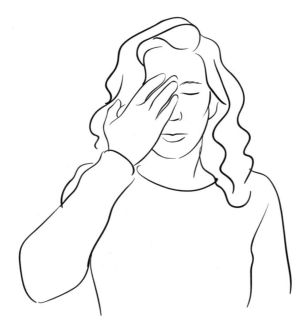

8. As you press on the third-eye point, feel a sense of calm wash over you with each exhale. Continue pressing for a minute or two.

9. Now move your middle finger to your *sternum* (breastbone) on the midline of your body, right between your breasts.

10. Press on the point on your sternum.

11. Again, feel a sense of calm with each exhale as you stimulate this calming point for a few minutes.

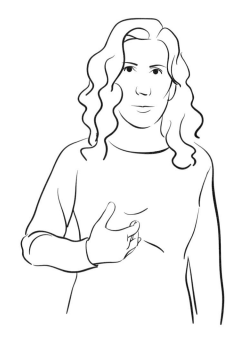

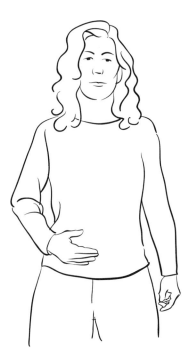

12. To end, place your middle finger about an inch directly below your navel. As you breathe, visualize breathing into and out of this point on your body. Feel yourself becoming grounded and rooted. This is the seat of your personal power, so feel yourself gaining control over your emotions while you focus on the point below your navel. Stay in that position for as long as you wish.

The visualizations during this exercise are very important. They will train your body to respond more quickly each time you practice. Pushing on the points assists your exhale in moving the anxiety downward through your body and then out through your feet. Note that you can always hold each point for a longer or shorter duration, depending on what your body and mind need at that time.

15. Acupoint Stimulation: For Digestion

This exercise helps you to digest a big meal, and it can also help to prevent chronic gas and bloating. As with the other exercises, the more you practice it, the more quickly you will see results. But in this case, you must also take an honest look at how you've been eating and see if there are ways to improve your eating habits. Even small changes add up, so I encourage you to find at least one change you can make to your diet, such as adding a salad to your lunch or dinner, or cutting out sodas in favor of green tea.

1. Sit upright in a chair and cross one leg over the other.

2. Use both hands to hold the big bone that runs down your leg from your knee to your foot (your *tibia*, or shinbone). About one inch away from the bone on both sides of your leg, apply pressure with all of your fingers. Your thumbs will be together on one side, and your fingers will be on the other side of your shinbone.

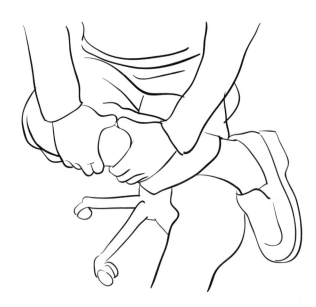

3. Squeeze your leg on both sides of the bone, beginning just below the knee. Knead and squeeze both sides of your leg and work your way down to your ankle. Take the time to stimulate the most sensitive areas along the way.

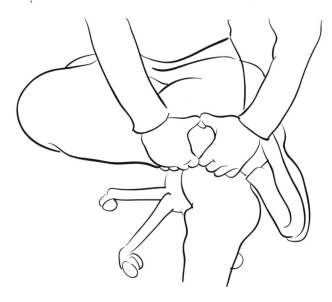

4. Work your way back up toward your knee, and then back down to your ankle again. Repeat at least 9 times up and 9 times down.

5. Switch legs by crossing the other leg over your knee. Apply pressure with all of your fingers to both sides of your leg about one inch away from either side of your shinbone.

6. Stimulate both sides of the shinbone at least 9 times down and 9 times up. 私

This exercise stimulates the spleen and stomach acupuncture channels, which are the channels most directly connected to the digestive process. Squeezing and rubbing the channels helps to move the qi to and from the digestive organs, thus aiding digestion and the peristaltic movement of food through your digestive tract.

16. Qigong Belly Rub: For the Bowels

This exercise is for constipation or diarrhea. It is especially good for people who suffer from irritable bowl syndrome or colitis. The nice thing about this exercise is that it can be customized. If you have constipation, you rub your belly in a circle along the pathway or flow of the large intestine. You rub the opposite way if you have diarrhea. If you would just like to keep things flowing smoothly, you can circle both ways.

I remember learning this exercise from a Chinese medicine master when I was still a student. He recommended that it be practiced every night before bedtime, or every morning before getting out of bed. Luckily, it can help any time it is practiced, but I still like to do it just before I get into bed. I find that focusing on my belly helps to move the energy out of my head, which helps me fall asleep more easily.

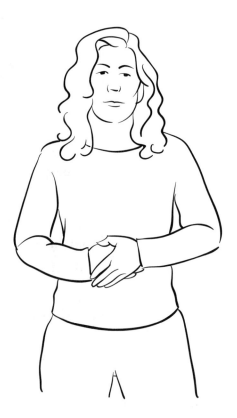

1. You can practice this lying down on your back, sitting upright in a chair, or standing in *wuji* posture.

2. Place one palm over your stomach (just below your *sternum*, or breast-bone), and place your other palm on the hand that is resting on your stomach.

3. For diarrhea, circle your entire abdomen counterclockwise, which means that you circle to the right, then down, then to the left past your navel, back up the left side of your body, and back to the starting position.

4. Repeat this circling movement 36 to 54 times, two to three times daily.

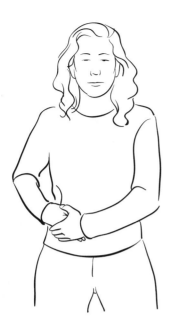
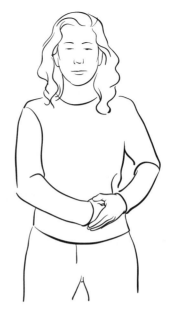

5. For constipation, you place your hands over your stomach as above, but this time you circle clockwise, which means you circle to the left, down the left side of your body, to the right just below your navel, back up the right side, and back to starting position. Repeat this circling movement 36 to 54 times, two to three times per a day.

6. As you circle, visualize a whirlpool forming in your abdomen from your belly to your back. See and feel the whirlpool circling in the direction your hands are circling, and feel your hands moving the whirlpool like magnetic energy.

7. If you would just like to keep your bowels moving smoothly, you can circle 36 times one way and then 36 times the other way, each time you do your daily practice.

Waste matter moves through your large intestine in a clockwise direction throughout your abdomen. The combination of intention and the movement of your hands sends a powerful message to your large intestine. This combination will help to regulate the movement of energy through your large intestine, which in turn affects the regularity of your bowel movements. This exercise is just too easy not to practice!

17. Healing Sound: For Heartburn

This is a simple exercise that makes use of sound vocalization to calm your stomach nerves and help bring your stomach back into balance. Emphasis is placed on the connection of mind, breath, and imagination to the area of focus. Sound vibrates through the body's internal cavities between the bones and within the organs, and that vibration helps to release stuck or stagnant qi, heat, and tension.

Heartburn and acid reflux can be caused by a variety of factors. For example, they can be due to bacteria, poor eating habits, and stress. The healing sound for heartburn helps to release stress from the stomach nerves and heat from the stomach. This exercise is particularly effective when combined with a healthy alkaline diet mostly consisting of vegetables, fruits, and grains.

The healing sound for heartburn and acid reflux is the *chu* sound (ironically, pronounced "chew!").

1. Stand in *wuji* posture or sit upright in a chair.

2. Rest your fingertips over your stomach, which is just below your *sternum* (breastbone). Hold your elbows slightly out so that your armpits are open.

3. Inhale a deep relaxed breath into your lower abdomen. Focus your mind on your stomach.

4. Exhale while you make the *chu* sound just by using your breath (as if you were whispering the sound) or by adding your voice to your breath.

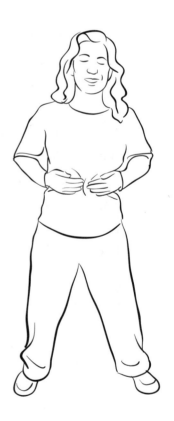

5. As you exhale the sound, feel your stomach relaxing and becoming cooler. Keep your mind focused on your stomach throughout this exercise.

6. Inhale into your lower abdomen, and then exhale the *chu* sound again, as it removes all the heat and tension from out of your stomach.

7. Repeat the sound 18 to 36 times, once or twice a day.

An alternate way to practice this exercise is to visualize the heat and acid from your stomach moving down to your legs, and then out through your feet, into the earth. Feel free to try both ways to discover which one is more powerful for you.

18. Qigong Lung Detox

This exercise stretches the lung tissue to help your lungs release toxins. It also helps to improve and increase your lung capacity so that you can take fuller, deeper inhalations. Breathing deeply is the cheapest and easiest form of detox there is, and the better you can do it, the better the detox. This exercise is perfect for people who are quitting smoking. It also helps lungs to heal and become stronger after an asthma attack, bronchitis, or a cold or cough.

1. Sit with your legs crossed. If you cannot sit on the floor, sit on a bed, a couch, or another suitable piece of furniture.

2. Place your hands directly down the sides of your body, with your palms resting on the floor.

3. Inhale fully and deeply through your nose while you turn your torso and head to the left, keeping your palms resting on the floor.

4. Hold your breath, turn to center, lean slightly forward, and exhale through your nose. Return to a straight spine

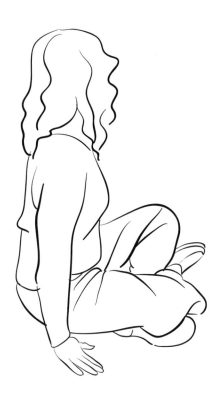

between this exhale and your next inhale.

5. Inhale while you turn your torso and head to the right.

6. Hold your breath, turn to the center, lean slightly forward, and exhale through your nose. Straighten your spine between that exhale and your next inhale.

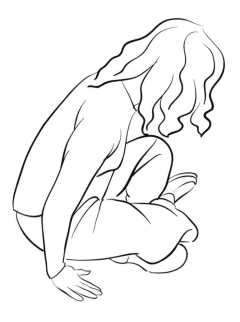

7. Always inhale while turning, and exhale while facing forward.

8. Repeat 18 to 36 times. 永

You don't have to be a smoker to practice this exercise; it is great for anyone who wants to strengthen her or his lungs. It feels like a movement meditation that strongly stretches and boosts lung qi. When practiced regularly, you'll find that this exercise is extremely calming to your emotions, which is indeed a large bonus.

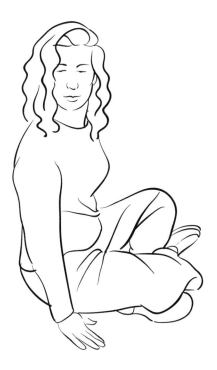

Foot Rub: For Insomnia

nia is one of the most common complaints I hear about from my patients. If you
don't sleep well or long enough, it can affect more than just your attention span and
energy. In fact, studies show that insomnia is associated with metabolic syndrome, a combination of physiological factors that leads to diabetes and heart disease (Gangwisch,
Heymsfield, and Boden-Albala 2006). Moreover, inadequate sleep throws off the regula-
tion of the hormones associated with hunger and satiety, which can cause obesity. Simply
stated, inadequate sleep can make you fat!

Many of us either have trouble turning our minds off or we fall asleep fine, but then
wake up too early and can't get back to sleep. This exercise helps to break those patterns.
It uses an acupuncture point on the foot, which is the first point on the kidney channel.
This channel helps to regulate the body's heat and fluids, which in turn helps to balance
your mind's awake and sleep cycles.

1. Just before bedtime, sit on the edge of your bed and cross one leg over the other.

2. Using the palm of your hand, vigorously rub the bottom of your foot from the heel to the ball and back. Rub at least 100 times as you visualize and feel the energy of your head, chest, and belly melting down to the bottom of that foot.

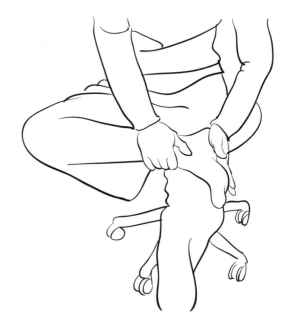

3. Switch feet and rub the bottom of the other foot vigorously at least 100 times, using the same melting visualization.

4. When you get into bed, lie on your back. Breathe slowly and deeply into and out of your belly.

5. When you exhale, visualize warm energy melting down from your head, through your torso, and going into and then out of your feet.

6. Repeat the visualization for 36 breaths.

In addition to practicing this exercise, I recommend that you not eat anything three hours before bedtime, and take a hot bath one hour before bedtime. After the bath, your temperature will drop, and that will help to make you sleepy. If you go to sleep with a full belly, your body is busy digesting, and it is harder for your body to fully rest, which means your mind won't get enough rest either.

20. Tongue Curl Breathing: For Weight Loss

This exercise is a meditation to aid your body to normalize hunger and fullness. As stated in exercise 19, a good night's sleep will help prevent weight gain. You also must make healthy changes to your eating habits for this exercise to have a beneficial effect.

Digestion begins in the mouth, and so you curl your tongue backward to inhibit the desire to eat. You also use your hands when you eat, and so your hands are also involved in this meditation. They are held in a *mudra* (hand posture) that helps to promote physical health and well-being.

1. Sit upright in a chair.

2. Place your hands on your thighs with your palms up, and touch your left ring finger to your left thumb, and your right ring finger to your right thumb.

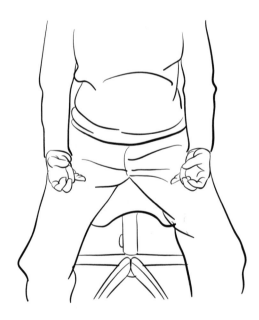

3. Begin abdominal breathing. Bring your attention to your belly and feel it expanding on the inhale and contracting on the exhale.

4. Curl your tongue up and then curl it toward the back of your mouth toward your throat. Make sure your tongue is comfortable, and don't push it so far back that you gag.

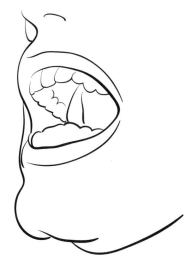

5. Continue abdominal breathing while focusing on your belly.

6. Feel a state of whole-bodied centered-ness and calm.

7. Practice this at least twice a day for three to five minutes each time. Try to work your way toward longer periods of meditation.

Meditation helps to keep you grounded and focused. When you are more centered, you are able to make better choices, including food choices. This exercise helps you to gain control over your cravings, and helps to put you in touch with your body, so that you are more aware of when you are truly hungry. This will help to stop you from eating when you are stressed or bored; that is, when your body is not sending out a true hunger signal.

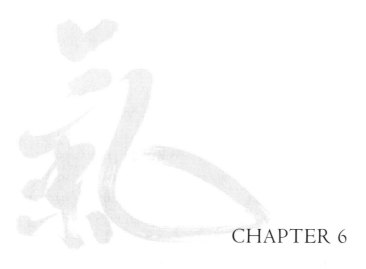

CHAPTER 6

BALANCING YOUR

EMOTIONS

Chinese medicine has recognized the body-mind connection for over two thousand years. The ancient theory of Chinese medicine views a person as composed of three inseparable parts: physical, energetic (which includes the emotions), and spiritual. Western medicine has always acknowledged the physical aspect of illness and, recently, has joined Chinese medicine in viewing the body and mind as inextricably linked, with both body and mind capable of affecting each other either positively or negatively. Health psychology, psychoneuroimmunology, and psychobiology are the three disciplines in Western medicine specifically dedicated to the study of the body-mind connection.

Controlled experiments carried out by allopathic doctors have strengthened the argument that the mind and the body can be used to heal each other. For example, studies have demonstrated that exercise is an antidepressant (Dunn et al. 2005), and that laughter boosts the strength of the immune system (Kamei, Kumano, and Masumura 1997).

Modern-day stress makes it difficult to maintain a healthy emotional balance. Today, many of us are on antianxiety or antidepressant medications. Although pharmaceuticals may help, they do not address *why* a person experiences certain feelings or how to cope with them, and they often come with unwanted side effects (like the inability to have an orgasm). I don't oppose the use of these drugs; they have their place and have saved many people from utter despair. However, the exercises in this section will provide you with natural and self-empowering ways to bring your emotions back into balance.

If you are on medication for an emotional or mood disorder, do not decrease the dose or discontinue taking it without the direct supervision of your doctor. I have used qigong to help patients reduce the number of their medications, or to get off their meds entirely, but only with the approval and help of their prescribing doctor.

These exercises help to bring your body into a calm and peaceful state, which in turn helps to calm your mind and emotions. Similarly, the calming visualizations use your mind to help relax the nerves of your body and to release tension and stress from your muscular system. Feel free to try just a few, many, or even all of the exercises in this section. Then continue to practice those that resonate most strongly for you. Or perhaps you should consider practicing the ones you are most resistant to, as a challenge.

You will be pleasantly surprised at how quickly you can develop the power to relax your body and mind in just a few minutes of practice a day.

1. Open Heaven and Close Earth: To Release Emotional Stress

I teach this exercise to all of my beginning qigong students. It's easy to learn and a very effective tool for getting out of your head and into your body. Circling your arms helps to relax the muscles of your chest and upper back, which are often tight due to stress. We tend to store and feel anxiety in our chests and our breathing patterns, and circling the arms helps the chest to open and release pent-up emotions, as well as muscular stress.

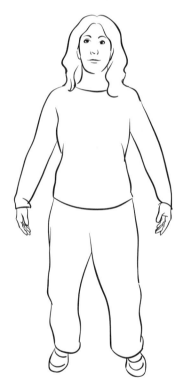

1. Stand in *wuji* posture. (You may sit in a chair, but standing is more powerful.)

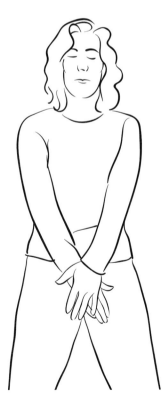

2. Place one palm over the back of your other hand, and let your arms hang down naturally in front of your body. Your hands should be at the midline of your body, approximately at the height of your groin.

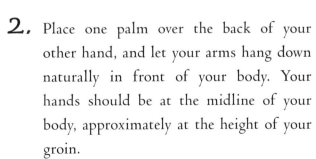

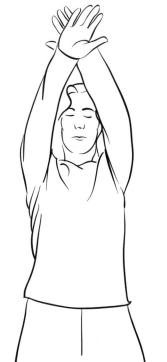

3. Inhale through your nose and into your abdomen as you raise your arms in front of you with your hands still together. Inhale until your hands are all the way above your head.

4. When your hands are above your head and still touching, exhale slowly through your mouth, and separate your hands and move your arms out to your sides as you lower them, making a big circle. That is, exhale while you lower your arms by stretching them out to your sides and "drawing" a big circle in a downward motion. After making the circle, rejoin your hands, one palm over the back of your other hand, just as you began this exercise.

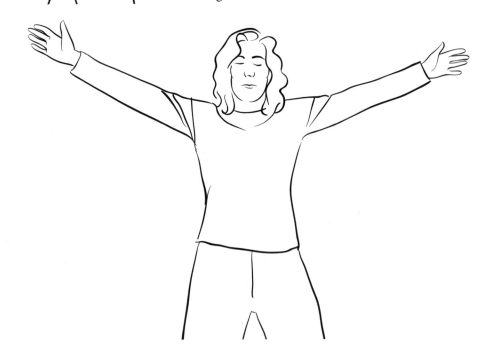

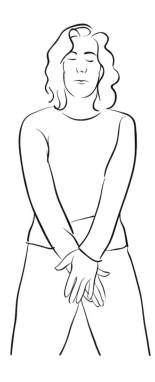

5. Place the palm of your other hand over the back of your hand, and repeat the exercise. Inhale while your hands are moving up in front of your body until they are above your head. Exhale as your hands move out to the sides of your body and back down to start again.

6. Repeat this exercise no fewer than 8 times. You can do sets of 8 repetitions until you feel relaxed and calm.

Breathing in through your nose fills your belly and lungs with fresh oxygen, which revitalizes your mind. Exhaling through your mouth helps to rid your body of toxins and is considered more sedating than exhaling through your nose. Exhale as if you are blowing through a straw. You can think of each exhale as blowing off steam! This exercise calms and soothes your nerves and initiates a deep relaxation response.

2. Flying Crane Spreads Its Wings: For Stress Reduction

If you frequently find yourself frustrated, impatient, or irritable, this is the exercise for you! It gives your physical body a way to release and expel pent-up stress, which will then help smooth the flow of your emotions. The arm movements help to relax your neck, arm, and upper back muscles, all of which become tight when you are stressed-out or burned-out.

   If your neck, upper back, or shoulders are stiff, you may find this exercise challenging at first. Luckily, if you practice it regularly, it will relieve that stiffness as it releases the tightness and tension from these areas, and the exercise will become easier.

1. Stand in *wuji* posture.

2. Bend your wrists so that your palms face the earth.

3. Inhale, bend your elbows, and raise your arms while keeping your wrists facing the earth. Be sure to keep your shoulders relaxed.

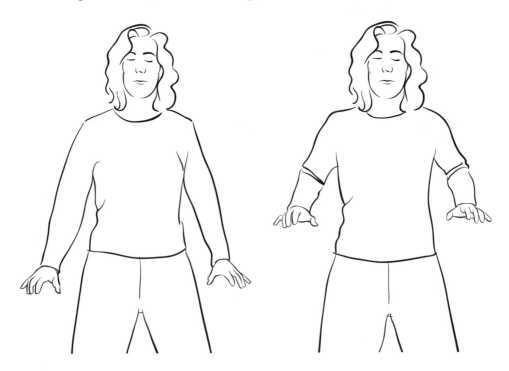

4. Exhale and push your arms back down, as if they were pressing something down into the earth.

5. Inhale and raise your arms again, and then exhale and push them back down.

6. Repeat one last time, for a total of 3 lifts and presses.

7. Before you inhale again, raise your hands in front of you to chest height with your elbows locked and your palms facing in the same direction you are facing. Your fingers point toward the sky.

8. Inhale, bend your elbows by dropping them down, and bring the backs of your hands toward your chest.

9. Exhale and slowly push your hands and arms back out to their outstretched position at chest height.

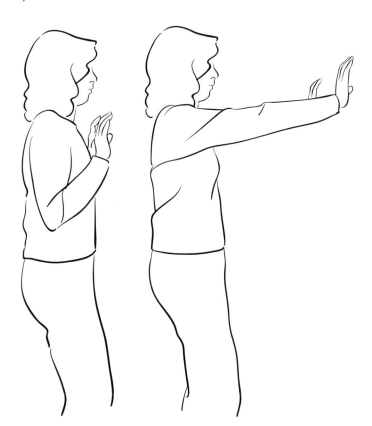

10. Repeat 2 more times. Be sure to breathe slowly and deeply with each movement.

11. Before your next inhale, rotate your arms out to the sides of your body with your palms at shoulder height (like a bird flapping its wings). Your wrists are bent and your fingers are pointing toward the sky.

12. Inhale while you drop your elbows and bring the backs of your hands toward your body at shoulder height.

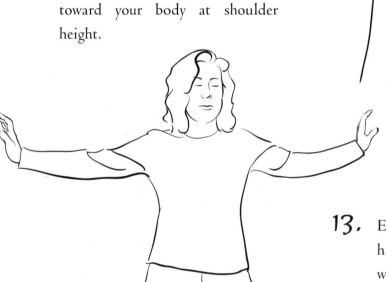

13. Exhale and push your hands away, as if you were pressing them against something, until your arms are fully extended out to your sides.

14. Inhale and bring your hands in toward your shoulders, and then exhale and push them back out to the sides.

15. Repeat one last time.

16. Before your next inhale, lower your hands to the original starting position, with your arms hanging down at your sides and your palms facing the earth. At this point, begin the entire set again; pushing toward the ground for 3 repetitions, pushing in front of your chest for 3 repetitions, and then pushing out to your sides for 3 repetitions.

There are two ways to enhance the benefits of this exercise. The first is to visualize pushing out anxiety, anger, irritability, stress, frustration, or any other negative emotion from your body when your hands are pushing away from your body. The second is to focus on coordinating your slow, deep breaths with slow, mindful hand movements. Whatever your focus, be sure to keep your shoulders relaxed throughout your practice. The slower you can practice this exercise, the bigger the release will be. This is an excellent stand-alone exercise when you need to release agitation.

3. Healing Sound: To Purge Anger and Stress

According to Chinese Five Element theory, the liver is the organ that stores anger and stress. In Western medicine, the liver is the organ that detoxifies blood. Chinese medicine holds that the liver also detoxifies your emotions so that they do not build up to a level of toxicity that can negatively affect your body functions.

1. Stand in *wuji* posture or sit upright in a chair.

2. Interlace your fingers and lift your hands over your head with your elbows straight, your fingers interlaced, and your palms facing the sky.

3. Tilt your torso to the left to open and stretch the area of the liver (which is located in the right side of your torso).

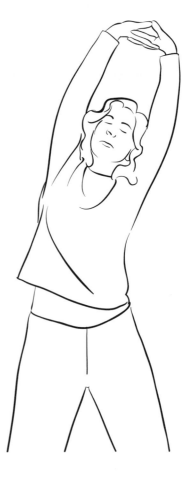

4. Inhale a deep relaxed breath into your lower abdomen. Focus your mind on your liver, which is under the lower part of your rib cage on your right side.

5. Exhale as you make the *shu* sound by just using your breath (as if you were whispering the sound) or by adding your voice to your breath.

6. As you exhale the sound, feel your liver releasing anger and stress from your whole body, coming out from your right torso area, as if your right torso were a magical

exit just for anger. Keep your mind focused on your liver throughout this exercise.

7. Inhale into your lower abdomen, and then exhale the *shu* sound again as it helps to release anger and stress from the area of your right torso, where your liver is located.

8. Repeat the *shu* sound 18 to 36 times, once or twice a day.

In qigong, the liver-healing sound is *shu* (pronounced "shoe"). The *shu* sound targets the liver and helps that organ to detoxify you both emotionally and physically. As with all healing sounds, you must focus your mind on the goal of the exercise to reap its benefits. For that reason, when you practice this exercise, you must find a way to visualize stress and anger being released from your liver, perhaps as a dark mist or a dense cloud of smog.

4. Healing Sound: To Purge Anxiety

Many of us store anxiety in our chest. When we do this, our anxieties produce the feeling that something rising up from our chest causes us to feel nervous, and it impedes our ability to take a deep breath. People who suffer from anxiety tend to be shallow breathers, although it is difficult to determine which came first. This exercise, along with most of the others in this book, utilizes slow, deep, abdominal breathing to help retrain the way we breathe so that our nervous system can relax.

Ha is the healing sound for anxiety; it is also the sound used to purge the sensations of emotional stagnation and heaviness from the heart and chest. We often release the *ha* sound unconsciously when we feel relieved. Therefore, we can bring ourselves emotional relief by using the *ha* sound consciously for therapeutic purposes.

1. Stand in *wuji* posture or sit upright in a chair.

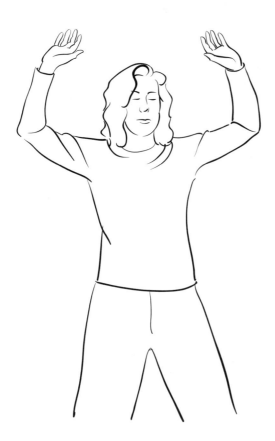

2. Raise your arms as if responding to someone saying "stick 'em up!" Your hands are a bit higher than your head and your palms face the direction you are facing. Keep your elbows slightly bent, and relax your shoulders.

3. Inhale a deep, relaxed breath into your lower abdomen. Focus your mind on the center of your chest between your breasts.

4. Exhale as you make the *ha* sound by just using your breath (as if you were whispering the sound) or by adding your voice to your breath.

5. As you exhale the sound, feel the anxiety being released out of your body, from your chest out through your mouth.

6. Inhale into your lower abdomen, and then exhale the *ha* sound again to release anxiety out through your mouth.

7. Repeat the sound either 8 or 16 times.

8. To end, place one palm on the center of your chest and one on your navel.

9. Take a few very slow abdominal breaths while visualizing your chest melting down into your abdomen.

Some people have a hard time holding their arms up during this exercise. This is usually due to neck and shoulder tension, both of which are common when you suffer from anxiety. Pay attention to how you are holding your shoulders; they should be relaxed and down. Rest assured that your arm, neck, and shoulder muscles will become stronger with practice, which will ease any discomfort you may have experienced initially. I encourage you to practice this exercise two or three times a day to speed up the release of long-term anxiety.

5. Healing Sound: To Purge Grief and Sadness

All of us have experienced grief and sadness in our lives. The question is not whether we have felt these emotions, but rather, what did we do with them? If we were able to fully enter our sadness and grief, then, eventually, whatever caused those feelings would become a memory from our past, triggered on occasion by certain reminders. However, if we were unable to fully experience the sadness and grief at the time they were appropriate, those emotions may have become stuck, or lodged in our consciousness. Now, we may find ourselves sad for no reason at all, or waves of sadness and grief may appear from out of the blue and dominate our moods without any specific memory triggers.

Sadness, which is said to be stored in the lungs, has the most direct effect on our breathing of any emotion. The way we breathe completely changes when we cry. Take a moment to try to initiate the breathing pattern that takes place when you cry, and you will understand what I mean immediately. The healing sound for sadness and grief is *shh*, which is the same sound parents make when trying to soothe a crying baby. In this instance, we use the sound to learn how to soothe ourselves.

1. Stand in *wuji* posture or sit upright in a chair.

2. Raise your elbows out to your sides at shoulder height. With your palms facing forward, tilt your forearms so that your fingers are pointing toward your head. Relax your shoulders. Do not bend your wrists.

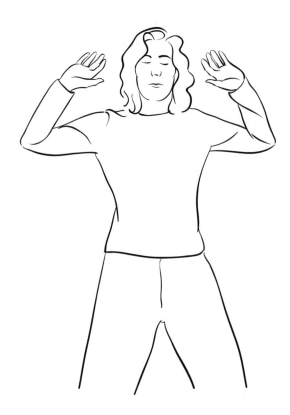

3. Inhale a deep, relaxed breath into your lower abdomen. Focus your mind on your lungs and under your entire rib cage: front, back and center.

4. Exhale as you make the *shh* sound just by using your breath (as if you were whispering the sound). As you exhale the sound, feel your lungs and chest releasing the sadness and grief from your whole body out through your mouth. Keep your mind focused on your lungs throughout this exercise.

5. Inhale into your lower abdomen, and then exhale the *shh* sound again, as it helps to comfort and soothe your sadness, and then releases the sadness through your mouth with each exhale. Allow the *shh* sound to make your body feel relaxed, heavy, and well grounded.

6. Repeat the sound 18 to 36 times, once or twice a day.

I like to prescribe this exercise to patients who are grieving a loss, or to those in psychotherapy dealing with chronic sadness. This is a good addition to talk therapy, since it helps to release grief directly from the body's tissues. However, if you are dealing with an intractable grief or an overwhelming sadness that prevents you from following a normal daily routine, you should first see a psychotherapist before beginning to work with this exercise.

6. Beating the Drum: For Focus and Concentration

This ancient exercise was used by Daoist masters to help improve mental focus during visualization meditations. It helps to clear what is commonly referred to as *brain fog*, or difficulty concentrating. Brain fog can occur when you are too exhausted to focus, or when you are juggling too many things at one time and are having a hard time keeping everything straight in your mind.

The "drum" in this exercise is the lowest part of the back of your skull. Many people have a small bump here, just above the area where the neck meets the head. This area of the brain is responsible for vision. You cover and close off your ears with your palms to keep out unwanted noise, and you turn your attention inward by closing your eyes. Thumping your fingers against this region of your head helps to clear your mind and invigorate your senses. It is a great way to feel refreshed when you have little time before your next appointment and you can't take a nap.

1. Stand in *wuji* posture or sit upright in a chair.

2. Rub your palms together vigorously until they become warm.

3. Place your palms over your ears with your fingertips resting on the back of your head, as if they were holding your head. Close your eyes for the remainder of the exercise.

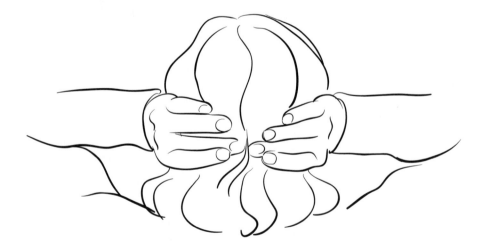

4. Press your index fingers on your middle fingers, and then bring your index fingers down onto your head with a "thump" sound. The middle fingers stay on the head while both index fingers move and make the "thump" sound at the same time as they hit the head.

5. Bring your index fingers back to press on your middle fingers again, and then let the index fingers gently hit your head again with a "thump."

6. Repeat the thumping sound 24 to 36 times slowly and rhythmically, like a pulse beat in your head.

7. Throughout this exercise, breathe slowly and deeply into your abdomen and relax your shoulders.

8. To end the exercise, pull your palms away from your ears with a quick movement, as if you were releasing suction cups, open your eyes, and take a deep breath.

I find that this practice helps me to clear my mind whenever I have too much on my plate, but I also use it to help get me sparked up when I feel too tired to focus. Try to experiment with the speed of the thumping to see if the effects of this exercise change for you the way they do for me. Also, it's easy to find yourself leaning forward when you do this exercise, so be sure to stay upright and to keep your shoulders relaxed.

7. Five-Element Visualization: For the Liver and Stress

Visualizations are great tools when you are in a public place and want to practice qigong without bringing attention to yourself. For example, this is a great exercise when you feel stressed-out during a meeting or when riding overcrowded public transportation.

As mentioned earlier, Chinese Five Element theory holds that green is the color for the liver, and the liver is the organ that stores stress. This visualization uses green imagery to direct your mind and attention away from stress.

1. Sit upright in a chair with your palms resting on your thighs. You can either close your eyes or lower them to look down in front of you.

2. Visualize yourself sitting safely in the middle of a dense forest, surrounded by green trees and plants, green foliage and leaves, and green ground cover. Take a few minutes to create an entire green environment in your mind's eye around you.

3. With each inhale, absorb the cooling, calming, grounding energy of the forest, like a green mist entering into your belly.

4. With each exhale, release all the stress and tension out of your body into the environment around you, where it is transformed into energy for the trees.

5. Continue to inhale the feeling of being in a forest, and to exhale your stress out into the green forest for as long as you wish. 气

Although this exercise seems very simple, its effects can be quick and profound. If you take just a few minutes to direct your mind toward something relaxing and stress free, you can step outside of your stressed-out feelings and thought processes. This is a way to create the space you need to change the way you think and feel in order to move toward living in a more balanced state of being.

8. Five-Element Visualization: For the Heart and Anxiety

Like exercise 7, this one is an excellent way to practice qigong without moving your body, making it perfect for practicing in public places. The previous exercise focused on stress reduction; this one is about releasing anxiety and calming your heart.

Although red is the Five Element color associated with the heart, it is considered too stimulating and heat inducing to work with during calming visualizations. So instead of the color red, we use the image of a sunrise, because both the sun and the morning are associated with the element of fire, along with the heart and the color red. We also touch our thumbs to our pinkies because the pinky is where the heart meridian ends.

1. Sit upright in a chair. Touch your left thumb to your left pinky, and your right thumb to your right pinky. You can either close your eyes or lower them to look down in front of you.

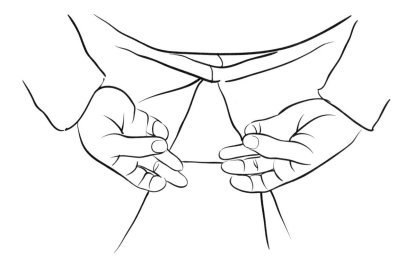

2. Visualize yourself sitting on a beach at sunrise. Take a few minutes to create the environment of an entire sunrise in your mind's eye.

3. See the red, orange, and yellow waves of light emanating from the rising sun. Watch the beach around you become more visible as the night recedes, and observe how the water reflects the colors of the sunrise. With each inhale, absorb the calming, gently warming rays of the sun into your body.

4. With each exhale, let the warmth melt all of your anxiety down through your body; let your anxiety flow from your chest on down, and then out of your body through your feet.

5. Continue to inhale the rising sun's rays, and exhale them to release and melt your anxiety down through your body and out through your feet, for as long as you wish.

Even though you are picturing the sun rising on the horizon, you will still visualize your anxiety moving down and out of your body in order to counteract the upward-moving nature of anxiety. Note that some people find that they become too warm during this exercise. If this happens to you, it may mean that you have too much heat in your body to begin with, and you should instead practice the healing sound to purge anxiety (exercise 4 in this chapter).

9. Waterfall Visualization: To Purge Stress

Let's face it: we can't always quiet our minds on command. Sometimes it is very hard to turn your mind off before beginning your qigong practice. There are days when even Cleanse the Qi, the first exercise in chapter 4, may not be enough to get you into the mood to practice. On such days, I like to begin with this simple visualization to help "wash me clean" of my racing thoughts so I can focus on the present moment. Think of this exercise as a "brain wash" to clear your mind of distracting thoughts and emotions.

1. Sit upright in a chair with your palms facing up on your thighs.

2. Visualize yourself sitting in a hot spring directly under a waterfall. Take a moment to create the environment in your mind's eye.

3. Visualize and feel the warm, or even slightly cool, water gently hitting your head and rolling down your neck, shoulders, back, and arms.

4. As you feel the water descending down your body, allow it to take all your racing thoughts, emotions, and physical tension down through and then out of your body.

5. Breathe deeply and slowly as you visualize and feel the water descending on your body, taking all your tension and stress with it.

6. Stay with the visualization as long as you wish, or until your mind and body feel calm and relaxed.

We use water to clean ourselves in the shower or bathtub, and we can also use images of water to clean ourselves off from whatever is preventing us from being fully present and relaxed. More often than not, it is our own minds or emotions that keep us from reaching a relaxed state in the midst of our busy and active lives. This visualization creates a virtual getaway so that you can cleanse yourself and be able to focus clearly and calmly on whatever comes next.

10. Rolling the Qi Ball: For Mental Focus and Centering

This meditative exercise is perfect for those times when it is hard to quiet your mind, or when you don't feel grounded and centered. I consider this exercise a "movement meditation," because it combines a meditative mental focus with simple meditative movements. If you always wanted to have a meditation practice but have had a hard time keeping your mind from wandering while meditating, this is the perfect exercise for you. I often recommend it to beginning meditators before they try to practice still meditations that require a quiet mind.

Note that this exercise was perfectly designed to practice at your desk at work for a quick, energy-refreshing, mind-clearing break.

1. Sit in a chair with your back straight and your feet firmly touching the ground.

2. Gently tuck in your chin to open the back of your neck. Drop and relax your shoulders. Keep your head directly centered above your torso.

3. Place your hands near your abdomen at navel height as if they were holding the sides of a full-sized basketball against your belly. Visualize that you are holding a ball of energy between your hands.

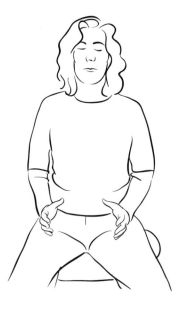

4. Inhale, and push the ball forward and then up to your chest height.

5. On your exhale, pull the ball in toward your chest and then back down to the original position in front of your belly.

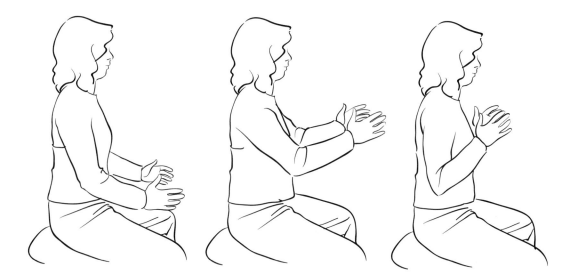

6. Your breath should be deep and as slow as possible while moving the ball in a continuous circle: forward and up with each inhale; in and down with each exhale.

7. With each inhale, feel your breath revitalizing and recharging your body with energy.

8. With each exhale, feel all your tension and worry sink down into your abdomen, away from your chest.

9. Begin with two to five minutes, twice a day, and work up to ten or fifteen minutes each time. 永

If you practice this exercise regularly, especially in the mornings, you will notice that you are more grounded and centered throughout your entire day. Once you are comfortable with this exercise, try to feel the energy between your hands as you roll the ball. Many people can feel the buildup of energy between their hands after a few minutes of practice. Try it to see if you are one of them.

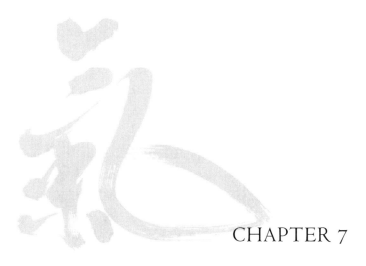

CHAPTER 7

CALMING YOUR SPIRIT

The word "spirit," when used in the context of Chinese medicine, is not connected with a religion or with any religious practices. Instead, it is seen as a reflection of our life force; of the quality of our lives, and of our will to live happily and healthily. A bright and vibrant spirit is reflected by balanced emotions and good physical health. Even after our bodies begin to break down from age-related causes, a strong spirit will continue to show in the brightness of our eyes and in the strength of our will.

Traditionally, you begin qigong training by strengthening your physical body. A strong body will provide you with the stamina for a long, productive practice. Once your body is in shape, you would then begin exercises that cleanse emotional sludge (which occurs when your emotions rule your moods) and to correct emotional imbalances so that you will have greater control over your reactions to emotionally charged events. Only after you have cultivated and refined your body and mind would you then turn your attention to the spirit. This makes good sense; if you are in a constant state of pain or emotional upset, it is much more difficult to access your spirit.

The next set of exercises will help you to access your spirit so that you can begin to program your thought patterns to be more honest with yourself and to have calmer reactions to the events in your life. You will be quieting your "monkey mind" (which is always racing from topic to topic) so that you'll feel what it's like to be in your body, and you can then deal with any emotional issues that warrant your attention. You can think of your spirit as your higher self; as that part of yourself that knows what is most beneficial for you and others. You can never fool or lie to your spirit.

The goal is to calm both your mind and body so that you can reach a state of peacefulness and tranquility. Many of the following visualizations focus on your physical body. They do that to help you improve your mental focus and to keep your mind from wandering. You will notice that after practicing any of these exercises on a regular basis, you will become more patient, more grounded, and more mindful.

You may find it helpful to record a visualization onto a tape or other device so you won't have to read while you are practicing. Reading while trying to meditate and visualize can be difficult, and it may even keep you from being fully present while you practice. Experiment to see what works best for you. Perhaps you have a friend with whom you can practice qigong, and you and your friend can take turns guiding each other through a meditation or two.

1. Sprouting Tree Roots: To Ground Mind and Body

Sometimes you just need something to get you out of your head—something that helps you to relax into your body. This tree-root visualization is a fabulous way to bring your consciousness down from your mind and into your feet. It is particularly helpful to practice this when you think you might lose your cool during a meeting or event scheduled later in your day. Practicing this exercise will root you like a tree and make you able to withstand even the strongest winds.

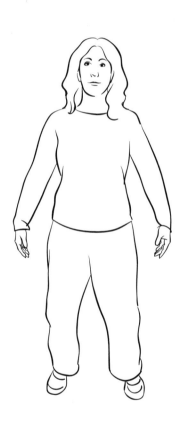

1. Stand in *wuji* posture or sit upright in a chair.

2. If you are seated, interlace the fingers of your left and right hands and let them rest comfortably in your lap.

3. Breathe slowly and deeply. With each inhale, fill your belly with energy, and with each exhale, let the energy sink down your legs and then into the ground. Practice this for a minute or two until your whole body begins to relax.

4. Now focus on your feet. Visualize your feet sprouting tree roots that go through the floor deep into the ground. In your mind's eye, watch them growing deeper and deeper into the earth. Take a full minute or even two to do this.

5. On an inhale, visualize pulling the grounding, centering earth energy up your tree roots, up your legs and thighs to fill your belly. You can visualize this as a golden mist rising from the earth's core into your belly.

6. Exhale, and visualize all your stress and worry exiting your body and melting deep into the ground through your tree roots.

7. With each inhale, pull grounding energy up through your tree roots, into your legs, and up to fill your belly. With each exhale, let all your tension and stress sink down into the earth's core via your tree roots.

8. Continue this meditation for as long as you wish.

The more regularly you practice this visualization, the more profound its effects. It can take ten minutes of practice every day to really feel the results of the practice, but once you do, you may soon be able to elicit the same response in a shorter period of time. I recommend using a golden color for the visualization, because yellow and gold are the colors associated with the earth and the earth element in Chinese Five Element theory.

2. Relaxation Visualization

Many of us go through the day without ever realizing how tense our muscles are. Mental stress can cause physical tension, but the opposite is also true; physical tension can make you mentally more tense and irritable. It's nice to take a few moments out of your schedule to check in and try to relax your entire body so that you can relax your mind. When your mind relaxes, it reinforces the relaxation in your body; this works like a positive feedback loop.

1. Sit upright in a chair with the backs of your hands resting on your thighs.

2. Breathe slowly and deeply into your belly.

3. Focus your attention on your head. Bring your awareness to the front, top, sides and back of your head. Get a good sense of how these areas feel.

4. Now visualize your head becoming heavier and heavier. On an exhale, visualize your head melting down into your chest. As it melts down, feel your neck completely relax.

5. Once you have felt your head melt into your chest, keep your awareness on your chest and upper back area. Focus on your front, the sides under your armpits, and your upper and middle back. Get a good sense of how they feel.

6. Now visualize your chest and back becoming heavier and heavier. On an exhale, visualize your chest and upper back melting down into your belly and low back. As they melt, feel your chest and upper back completely relax.

7. Once your chest and upper back have melted into your belly and low back, bring your attention and awareness to your belly, sides, and low back. Get a good sense of how each body part feels.

8. Now visualize your belly and low back becoming heavier and heavier, until they melt down through your knees and into the earth. As they melt into the ground, they take with them any tension left in your torso and knees.

9. Take a few moments to focus on your breath before concluding this exercise.

This is a great way to begin or end your qigong practice. You can also try to find a quiet time every day to do this. No matter when you practice this visualization, you will feel all of your muscles relax, and that deep relaxation will flow into your mood.

3. Gathering Earth Energy

Why try to visualize gathering energy from the earth? Because according to Chinese medicine theory, the earth's energy is very grounding, rooting, calming, and cooling. It is powerful enough to support the growth of plants, vegetables, and trees—all of which send their roots deep into the earth for nourishment.

This exercise helps to counteract the effects of being too active and running around too much day after day. Constant activity without any rest is said to send everything in an upward direction, such as our blood pressure, our anger, and our anxiety. If you finally do get the chance to rest or sleep and you can't, this exercise is for you.

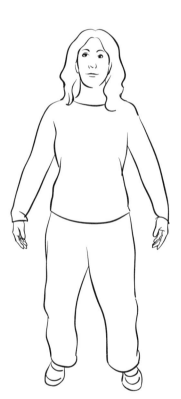

1. Stand in *wuji* posture or sit upright in a chair.

2. Let your hands hang loosely at your sides and your fingertips point toward the ground.

3. Bring your attention and awareness to your hands.

4. Visualize them growing longer and sinking down into the ground beneath you. If you are indoors, let them sink through the floor into the earth beneath you.

5. Visualize the feeling of the ground in your hands. Take a moment to consider the texture of the earth that lies beneath you (or the floor if you are indoors).

6. Now visualize the calming, cooling, grounding energy of the earth traveling up your elongated hands, through your arms, and into your chest. The energy should be sucked up into your body in the way that a straw sucks up liquid from a glass.

7. Take as long as you need to feel the earth's grounding energy fill your feet, then legs, groin, waist, belly, chest, arms, and all the way up to your head.

8. Feel your body vibrating with the earth's calming energy from your feet up to your head.

9. Take a few deep breaths before concluding this meditation.

This is a great exercise to practice outdoors, especially on the grass or a beach. We all spend so much time indoors; this meditation gives you a great reason to step outside and take a few minutes for yourself. It will refresh and recharge you when you are feeling rushed and burned-out. You may feel heavier (in a positive, grounded way), or you may feel as though you need to move more slowly. Great! Slower still gets you there, but without the stress.

4. Gathering Heaven (Environmental) Energy

Chinese texts use the word "heaven" to refer to the sky and everything in it. I sometimes use the phrase "the sun, the moon, and the stars" instead of the word "heaven" to avoid any unintentional religious connotations. As opposed to the grounding, calming energy of the earth, heaven's energy is considered more active and stimulating.

This next exercise is designed to give you an energy recharge when you are feeling tired. However, it is not for those times when you are tired from lack of rest or lack of sleep; in those instances only rest and sleep will do. It is for when you have an afternoon crash and you need to be alert and focused for the next few hours. Although you can do this in a seated position, you will get a bigger charge if you practice while standing, which is more helpful for circulating blood and waking you up.

1. Stand in *wuji* posture or sit upright in a chair.

2. Bring your arms up and straight out to your sides at shoulder height, with your palms facing the sky. Don't bend your elbows, but be sure to relax your shoulders.

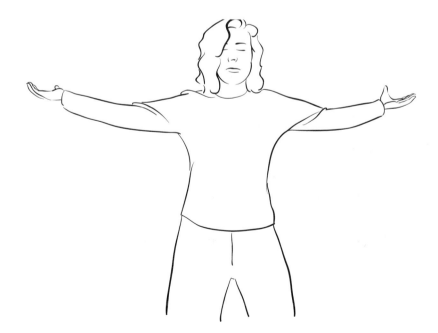

3. Inhale, and bring your arms up straight up above your head, with your palms still facing the sky and your fingertips now pointing toward each other. Try to keep your arms as straight up as possible; you may need to bend your elbows a little for comfort. Relax your shoulders.

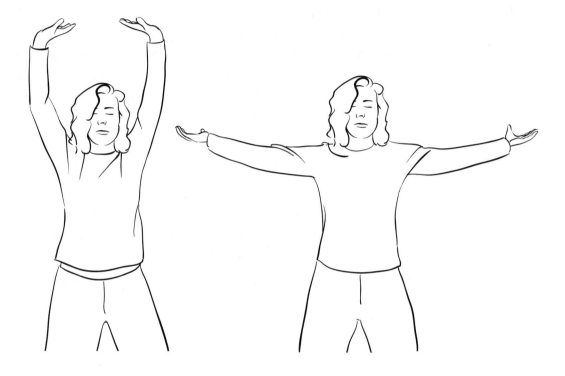

4. Exhale, and bring your arms back out to your sides with your palms still facing up.

5. Inhale as you bring your hands up above your head, as straight as is comfortable. As you inhale, visualize gathering the stimulating energy of the sky above with your hands and moving it into your body.

6. As you exhale, bring your hands down to shoulder height, and visualize and feel the stimulating energy of the sun, moon, and stars fill and energize your whole body.

7. Repeat for a total of 9 or 18 times.

It is important to remember to breathe fully and deeply into your belly during this exercise. The deep breaths will bring much-needed oxygen to your cells, which will use that oxygen to make more energy. Move your arms in sync with your deep breathing. Your hands remain facing the sky and move as if carrying something on a plate. Your shoulders may want to move up when you raise your arms; try to keep them down and relaxed.

5. Spontaneous Qigong Bliss

This style of qigong became very popular in China in the 1980s, and it now has quite a following in the United States. *Spontaneous* qigong is the practice of allowing your body to move without planning the movements. Rather than follow a step-by-step exercise routine, you simply observe which parts of your body want to move, and where and how they want to move, and then you let them do it. Although this can be fun to watch (and let me tell you it is fun!), the practitioner finds it very cathartic and soothing.

You will want plenty of room and privacy when you first practice this free-flowing style of qigong. If you are self-conscious, you will be unable to sense and respond to your body's natural flows and rhythms, so a comfortable atmosphere is essential. Some people like to put music on to practice with, so find a piece of music that you really enjoy to help you get into the mood. Then, just go with your flow. Here are some tips to get you started:

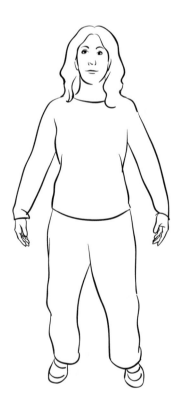

1. Stand in *wuji* posture and practice a few repetitions of Cleanse the Qi (exercise 1 in chapter 4).

2. Continue to practice Cleanse the Qi until you feel as though your arms want to move in a different way, and then let them do it.

3. Allow your arms to twist your torso so that you are also moving your waist.

4. Take a step forward to the side, or backward, and see how that step changes your hand and waist movements.

5. Move your other foot and see how that changes the rest of your movements.

6. At some point, add your neck and head to your moves. Move, twist, and bend your head, which will then pull your shoulders in new directions.

7. Continue for at least five minutes, or until the music ends.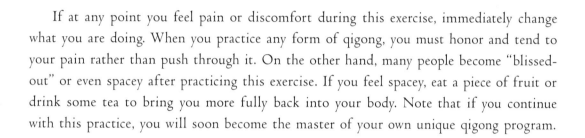

If at any point you feel pain or discomfort during this exercise, immediately change what you are doing. When you practice any form of qigong, you must honor and tend to your pain rather than push through it. On the other hand, many people become "blissed-out" or even spacey after practicing this exercise. If you feel spacey, eat a piece of fruit or drink some tea to bring you more fully back into your body. Note that if you continue with this practice, you will soon become the master of your own unique qigong program.

6. Buddhist Greeting Pose for Tranquility

The traditional Buddhist greeting involves placing your hands in prayer position and then bowing to the person whom you are greeting, who then repeats the same gestures. Interestingly, the acupuncture meridian for the heart runs down the arms into the palms. When you place your palms together, you are sealing energy into your heart and heart meridian. It is as though the Buddhists make a heart-to-heart greeting to each other when they meet, and their hands are indeed held directly in front of their hearts.

In qigong practice, we use this posture to calm the heart, which also means to calm the emotions. It is a simple meditation to take you out of your environment and into your own body and mind, which is perfect when you feel as if you've been too busy to hear your own thoughts. The calm you begin to feel is practically instantaneous.

1. Sit upright in a chair.

2. Place your palms together in prayer position in front of your chest.

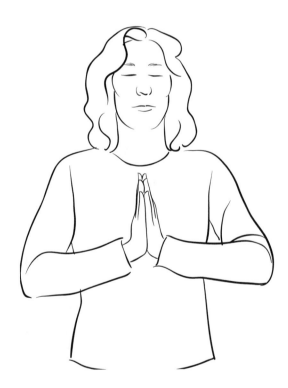

3. Breathe slowly and deeply into your belly.

4. Place your attention on your chest and upper back while you breathe.

5. Feel your chest and back relax with each inhale and exhale.

6. Feel waves of calm spread from your chest and upper back to the rest of your body.

7. Continue focusing on the calm spreading throughout your body for as long as you wish. 私

You can practice this exercise for ten minutes, or you may do it for only three minutes. Either way, you are sealing off your heart so that it can relax into the present moment, free from any distractions. When your heart is relaxed, you have a better grasp on your emotions and your mood. Learn from the wisdom of the Buddhist sages.

7. Energy-Bubble Visualization

People often ask me if there is a qigong exercise to help protect them when they are about to enter an uncomfortable situation. For example, sometimes they want an exercise they can do before, during, and after they visit their families. Sometimes they want to prepare for a big meeting. And sometimes they just want something they can do before they go to work each day. Interestingly, the doctors who practice ancient Chinese medicine use this type of visualization before they work with contagious patients, in the same manner that surgeons wear gloves and masks.

Energy-bubble visualizations work because you invest your valuable time and energy in creating a protective space surrounding you that cannot be invaded without your permission. When you invest this time and energy, your body becomes programmed with the message you are creating. If you decide that you won't allow someone to knock you off your center and you take steps to prevent it, you minimize the chance of it happening.

1. Stand in *wuji* posture or sit upright in a chair with the backs of your hands resting on your thighs (palms up).

2. Close your eyes and slow your breathing. Feel your whole body relax.

3. Visualize a bubble around your body in your mind's eye. Take as much time as you need to mentally create a thick bubble enveloping you. Visualize and "see" the shape, color, and size of the bubble.

4. Once you clearly see yourself surrounded by a bubble, draw up a memory of a time or an experience when you felt particularly powerful, calm, or in charge.

5. Let that feeling emanate out of your body to fill the entire bubble. Take a minute or two to do this. Perhaps the feeling has a color or quality you can see that fills the bubble.

6. After you've filled your bubble, take another minute to see and feel it surrounding you.

7. Take a few deep breaths before concluding this meditation.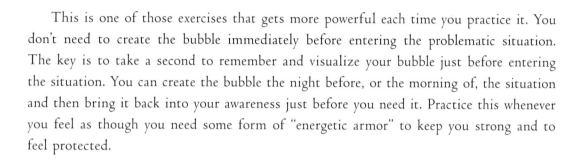

This is one of those exercises that gets more powerful each time you practice it. You don't need to create the bubble immediately before entering the problematic situation. The key is to take a second to remember and visualize your bubble just before entering the situation. You can create the bubble the night before, or the morning of, the situation and then bring it back into your awareness just before you need it. Practice this whenever you feel as though you need some form of "energetic armor" to keep you strong and to feel protected.

8. Inhaling the Calm

This exercise is a great breathing technique to use if you have tried to meditate but can't seem to keep your mind from racing from one thought to the next. I frequently teach this in classes because it is easy to learn and profoundly relaxing. This breathing technique works by sinking stress and tension down and away from the chest area. You are then taken into a much more peaceful and relaxed state of being.

1. Sit upright in a chair with your fingers interlaced and your hands resting together in your lap.

2. Focus on your belly. Inhale slowly and push your belly out, and then exhale slowly and pull your belly in. Take a few breaths while focusing on your belly.

3. On an inhale, visualize a silver ball of energy being inhaled into your chest.

4. On the exhale, visualize and feel the ball of energy sink into your belly.

5. Remember, as your belly pushes out, you inhale an energy ball into your chest. As your belly pulls in, the energy ball sinks into your belly.

6. Try to keep your mind focused on the energy ball coming into your chest and sinking down into your belly.

7. Repeat this breathing pattern and notice how your body and mind relax into the movements of your belly.

8. Continue this exercise for three to ten minutes.

This is yet another one of the exercises that can be practiced in public places without bringing attention to yourself. Try to find a nice spot in your backyard, a nearby park, or somewhere in nature, and see what it is like to inhale the calm of that special place.

9. Fire in the Belly

Think of this exercise as a qigong bio-battery boost. Heat is a form of energy, and when you visualize fire somewhere inside of yourself, you bring more heat and energy to that region. With regular practice, you will be able to feel the area below your navel become warm or heavy with the sensation of energy.

Your abdomen is considered the residence of your "energetic gas tank" (called lower *dantien* in Chinese, or your "core" if you do Pilates work). This exercise uses visualizations to add fuel to the fire in your belly, to help with moving forward in life and with making decisions from your gut. Bringing your attention to your low belly will divert it from your mental chatter, which will have a calming effect on your entire nervous system. This exercise is therefore energizing as well as calming.

1. Sit upright in a chair with your left thumb touching your left ring finger, and your right thumb touching your right ring finger. Your hands can rest on your thighs. Feel free to close your eyes.

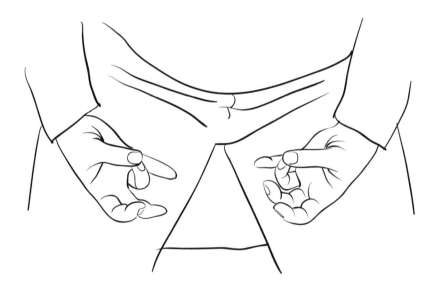

2. Slow your breath and quiet your mind.

3. Focus your attention on the whole area of your belly below your navel. Imagine a ball of fire located within your torso, just behind and below your navel.

4. As you breathe into and out of your belly, visualize the fire burning in your low abdomen. Keep your attention on the shape, size, and colors of the fire.

5. If your mind begins to wander, bring it back to the fireball inside of your abdomen.

6. Continue to focus on your fire until you feel refreshed and energized.

You touch your thumbs to your ring fingers during this exercise because your ring fingers represent the region of your lower belly. You use your hands to help bring even more attention to that region, which will support your visualization. This is the kind of exercise that grows on you; at first, it seems simple and maybe even a little bit boring, but it really does feel as if you are being recharged while you also rest in the stillness.

10. Third Eye Connection Meditation

The third eye is considered the seat of your intuition, your higher self, and of "knowing without knowing." This exercise helps connect you to this region and therefore to your spirit and higher self. There is an acupuncture point above the bridge of your nose between your eyebrows, exactly where your third eye would be. I use that acupoint, called *yintang*, on almost every patient because it elicits a strong relaxation response. This exercise teaches you how to stimulate that point by yourself, and then focus on the point to gain greater clarity of mind.

1. Take a fingernail and gently press the area above your nose between your eyebrows—the area of your third eye. Then, rub that spot in small circles first to the right and then to the left.

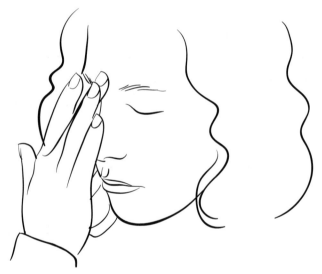

2. Once you can still feel the point on your face without your finger there, interlace your fingers and rest your hands in your lap. Close your eyes.

3. As you practice abdominal breathing, keep your awareness on the sensations of your third eye. With your eyes still closed, you can gently turn your eyes toward the third eye point—but do not strain to do so.

4. Visualize a light in the area of your third eye. As you sit there breathing, notice the light slowly becoming brighter and brighter. Take a few minutes to watch the light grow stronger and stronger until it fills your entire head.

5. When the light is at full brightness, visualize it sinking like the sun or moon, down from your head and into your belly.

6. You can begin this exercise again by stimulating your third eye point with your finger before focusing on the area, or you can conclude your practice here.

It is very important to sink the bright light down from your head and into your belly when you end this exercise. If you already have too much energy in your head, as evidenced by headaches, for example, you may bring on a headache if you leave the bright light in your head instead of sinking it below, into your belly. This exercise will help to clear out any brain fog or fuzzy thinking; it is an excellent practice to follow before making important decisions.

11, Gratitude Meditation

Sometimes we just need to take a step back and reassess what is happening in our lives. Are things really so bad? If they are, what can you do about it? Or, if you feel stuck or helpless, what are the positive things, the highlights, of your days that you can focus on to keep you going? No matter how hard life may seem to be, we all have something for which we are grateful. It could be a loved partner, an amiable coworker, a beloved pet, your home, your garden, your music collection—whatever brings you joy when you think about it.

I like to practice this exercise after I realize that I've been freaking out over something that will seem quite trivial once it is over with or finished. It helps to bring me perspective and gets me focused on the things in my life that matter and that deserve the attention I am wasting on something trivial and fleeting. Practice this and you'll know exactly what I mean.

1, Sit comfortably in a chair with your hands resting on your thighs, palms up, or lie on your back with your arms and legs splayed out comfortably, like a gingerbread person or a snow angel. If you are lying down, turn your palms up to face the sky.

2, Slow your breath and quiet your mind.

3, Get a sense of how your body feels. Is it tense? Relaxed? Can you bring some relaxing energy to the tense areas? Take a few moments to really feel your body, from the top of your head to the bottoms of your feet. Don't judge how you feel; just feel.

4, Now think of something in your life that you are grateful for, or something you are grateful to have had or experienced in the past. Pull up an image or a memory, and then let the accompanying feelings of gratitude fill your entire being.

5, Feel the waves of gratitude energize every cell in your body, from your head to your toes and then back up, from your toes to your head.

6. Stay with that image, or pull up another image of something or someone for whom you are grateful. Let that sense of gratitude fill and energize every cell in your body.

7. You can continue to make a gratitude list in your head, or stop at just one image.

8. When you feel that you have been completely recharged with your gratitude, take a few deep breaths before concluding this exercise.

You have the option of thinking of one image each time you practice this, or of making a list of the things for which you are grateful. Even if you have only one thing you can think of, if it is meaningful for you, it can always be used to change your mood and mind-set.

12. Manifestation Meditation

This is the only exercise in the book that involves mantra practice. You may have heard the word "mantra" in a yoga or meditation class. It means a word or a phrase that is repeated over and over to help you with concentration and spiritual intention. You can repeat a mantra out loud, or silently in your head. It is one way to focus your mind and energy toward a specific goal, whether spiritual or material.

There are plenty of books and movies about manifesting your dreams, many of which read like qigong theoretical manuals. They are based on the concept that we bring about what we think about, or that we send out thought vibrations that attract certain people or events to us. It is as if we are radios, and we pick up some signals better than others, and we put out stronger or weaker signals at different times.

You should honestly assess your goals and desires before beginning this exercise. The question to ask yourself is whether the change you want to happen will bring you true happiness, or whether it is a Band-Aid you might use to cover up an issue that needs to be addressed. Once you know what you want in your life, when you are really clear, this meditation will help to change your "radio frequency" to one that more easily receives and manifests your dreams.

1. Find a piece of paper and a writing utensil. Make them both special; for example, use fancy stationery paper and a brightly colored magic marker or your favorite pen.

2. Write "Thank you for" or "I give thanks for" on your paper, and then fill in what it is that you would like to have happen. Write only one sentence or phrase giving thanks for having achieved your goal or desire.

3. Take a look at what you wrote and examine how you wrote it. If you are not satisfied, rewrite it the way you want to see it.

4. Place the paper somewhere special, such as on an altar or in a special place in your bedroom or office.

5. Sit upright in a chair with your fingers interlaced and resting in your lap.

6. Slow your breath and relax your mind.

7. Repeat the sentence, which is your mantra, slowly and mindfully. You may do so aloud, in a whisper, or silently inside your mind.

8. Imagine your words rippling out into the environment around you as you repeat them. Take a few minutes to slowly repeat your mantra and feel the words ripple out all around you.

9. Release the ripples of your mantra out into the universe before concluding your meditation.

When you write the thank-you note, you write it as if your desire has already come true. Manifestation is more powerful when you truly believe that you have already received what you wanted, and that it is just a matter of time before you see it with your own two eyes. Writing down your mantra gives even more energy to your dream, as you are forced to put your thoughts into concrete, tangible, touchable words.

It is fitting to end this qigong book with a manifestation meditation, as the practice of qigong itself manifests health, happiness, and longevity. If you practice any one of these exercises consistently and diligently even for just a few minutes every day, you will start to see results more quickly than you might imagine.

There is a famous saying "Where the mind goes, the qi follows." If you focus your attention and intention during an exercise, your body's energy will respond accordingly. Above all else, you should enjoy your practice. Health and healing come quicker with a smile than with a furrowed brow! May your qigong practice bring you double happiness. Good luck!

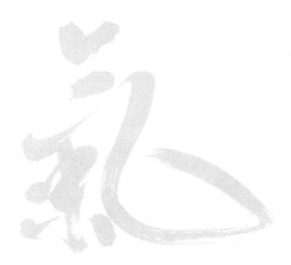

RECOMMENDED READING

Chan, Luke. 1999. *101 Miracles of Natural Healing*. West Chester, Ohio: Benefactor Press.

Chuen, Lam Kam. 1999. *Chi Kung: The Way of Healing*. New York: Broadway Books.

Cohen, Kenneth S. 1997. *The Way of Qigong*. New York: Ballantine Books.

Helms, Joseph M. 2007. *Getting to Know You*. Berkeley, CA: Medical Acupuncture Publishers.

Kohn, Livia (ed.). 2006. *Daoist Body Cultivation*. Magdalena, NM: Three Pines Press.

Kohn, Livia (ed.). 1989. Gymnastics: The ancient tradition. In *Taoist Meditation and Longevity Techniques*. Ann Arbor: Center for Chinese Studies, the University of Michigan.

Liu, Hong, with Paul Perry. 1997. *The Healing Art of Qi Gong*. New York: Warner Books Inc.

O'Connor, Dermot. 2006. *The Healing Code*. London, England: Hodder Headline Ireland.

Oleson, Terry. 1996. *Auriculotherapy Manual*. Los Angeles, CA: Health Care Alternatives.

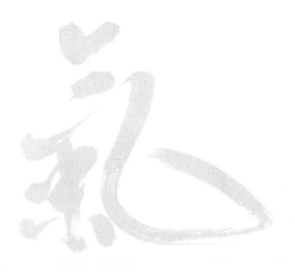

REFERENCES

Curiati, J. A. 2005. Meditation reduces sympathetic activation and improves the quality of life in elderly patients with optimally treated heart failure: A prospective randomized study. *Journal of Alternative and Complementary Medicine* 11(3):465-72.

Dunn, A., M. H. Trivedi, J. B. Kampert, C. G. Clark, and H. O. Chambliss. 2005. Exercise treatment for depression: Efficacy and dose response. *American Journal of Preventive Medicine* 28(1):1-8.

Gangwisch, J. E., S. B. Heymsfield, and B. Boden-Albala. 2006. Short sleep duration as a risk factor for hypertension: Analyses of the first National Health and Nutrition Examination Survey. *Hypertension* 47(5):833-839.

Kamei T., H. Kumano, and S. Masumura. 1997. Changes in immunoregulatory cells associated with psychological stress and humor. *Perceptual and Motor Skills* 84:1296-1298.

Lee, A., and M. L. Done. 1999. The use of nonpharmacologic techniques to prevent post-operation nausea and vomiting: A meta-analysis. *Anesthesia & Analgesia*, online journal of the International Anesthesia Research Society. www.anesthesia-analgesia.org/cgi/content/abstract/88/6/1362.

Myeong, S. L., K. H. Yang, H. J. Huh, H. W. R. Kim, H. S. Lee, and H. T. Chung. 2001. Qi therapy as an intervention to reduce chronic pain and to enhance mood in elderly subjects: A pilot study. *American Journal of Chinese Medicine* 29(2):237-245.

Peng, H. 1990. A primary study on the Han bamboo strip gymnastic book from the Han bamboo strips of Zhangjiashan. *Wenwu* vol. 10: Beijing, China.

Rossman, M. L. 2000. *Guided Imagery for Self-Healing*. Novato, CA: New World Library.

Sancier, K. M. 1996a. Anti-aging benefits of qigong. *Journal of the International Society of Life Information Sciences* 14(1):12-21.

———. 1996b. Medical applications of qigong. *Alternative Therapies in Health and Medicine* 2(1):40-46.

Sancier, K. M., and D. Holman. 2004. Commentary: Multifaceted health benefits of medical qigong. *Journal of Alternative and Complementary Medicine* 10(1):163-166.

Tsang, W. H., C. K. Mok, Y. T. Au Yeung, and S. Y. C. Chan. 2003. The effect of qigong on general and psychosocial health of the elderly with chronic physical illnesses: A randomized clinical trial. *International Journal of Geriatric Psychiatry* 18(5):441-449.

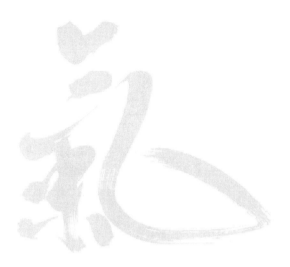

Suzanne B. Friedman, L.Ac., DMQ (China), is an acupuncturist, herbalist, and doctor of medical qigong therapy. Friedman is the first non-Chinese person to be inducted into her teacher's lineage as a Daoist qigong master. She is chair of the Medical Qigong Science Department at the Acupuncture and Integrative Medicine College in Berkeley, CA. Friedman is clinic director of Breath of the Dao, a Chinese medicine clinic in San Francisco, CA. Her articles on qigong and Daoism have appeared in numerous journals and magazines nationwide.